PMS: *The legends*
Menstruating women have the power to sour
wine, blight crops and ruin mirrors . . . each
month they become dangerous and unpredict-
able, witchlike bearers of the mysterious, magical "curse."

PMS: *The facts*
Many, perhaps most, women suffer from a variety of symptoms associated with the menstrual
period—among them tension, depression, swelling and anger. Many suffer from pain that ranges
from mild to excrutiating. *But this condition—*
PMS—is physical in origin and is treatable by
simple, natural means.

In this authoritative book, Carlson Wade offers a look at
the progress in PMS research that has finally demysti-
fied the condition, and the new multi-faceted natural
program that has brought relief and new hope to millions of PMS sufferers everywhere.

CARLSON WADE'S

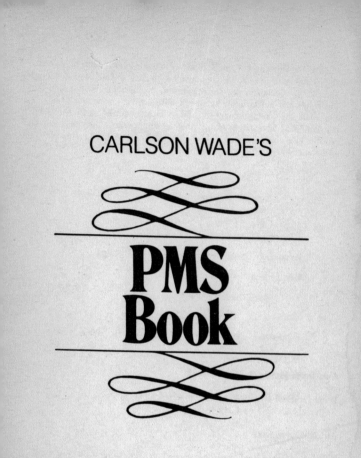

PMS Book

Keats Publishing, Inc. New Canaan, Connecticut

Carlson Wade's PMS Book

Pivot Original Health Edition published 1984

Copyright © 1984 by Carlson Wade

Library of Congress Catalog Number: 84-80808

ISBN: 0-87983-371-8

Printed in the United States of America

PIVOT ORIGINAL HEALTH BOOKS are published by

Keats Publishing, Inc.
27 Pine Street (Box 876)
New Canaan, Connecticut 06840

Contents

Chapter 1

THE MYTHS OF MENSTRUATION

THROUGHOUT THE AGES, many societies have labelled menstruating women "unclean." Others have considered them to be dangerous. Superstition was so strong in some societies that it was believed entire cattle herds would perish if they came close to a woman who was in the midst of her "unclean" period. Women in certain tribes were instructed to keep out of the sight of the men, and never to touch garments, eating utensils or sleeping mats that were to be used by the men for fear that contamination would cause a plague. Even today, menstruating women are declared taboo in certain societies.

Menstruation is a perfectly natural and healthy process, but for many it is still shrouded in mystery; that is why PMS is much in the news. Certain myths still linger that make many women (and men) apprehensive and even fearful of this biological process.

The Greek philosopher Aristotle (384-322 B. C.) declared that "the glance of a menstrual woman takes the polish from a mirror and the person who next glances in it will be bewitched." This view was shared by the Roman philosopher Pliny the Elder (23-79 A. D.) in his *Natural History*, where he cautioned that uncovering

1

the body of a menstruating woman gave her the power
to stop lightning, whirlwinds and hailstorms: "Nothing
could easily be found that is more remarkable than the
monthly flux of women. Contact with it turns new wine
sour, crops touched by it become barren, grafts die,
seeds in gardens are dried up, the fruit of trees falls off,
the bright surfaces of mirrors in which it is merely
reflected is dimmed, the edge of steel and gleam of
ivory are dulled, hives of bees die, even bronze and
iron are at once seized by rust, and a horrible smell
fills the air: to taste it drives dogs mad and affects their
bite with an incurable poison."

According to beliefs attributed to Aeolus, the Greek
god of the winds, a woman in the midst of her monthly
period was also in direct contact with the stars and
possessed magical powers.

All these superstitions may have arisen for one simple reason. Ancients looked upon the monthly bleeding
cycle as something magical: a woman could go through
this process without dying. She obviously had a mysterious ability to bleed and then recover . . . month after
month. The primitives did not seem to notice the fact
that women did not bleed when pregnant or breast-
feeding. Nor did they seem to notice that animals bled,
too, when in the throes of heat.

The noted gynecologist Niels H. Lauersen, M.D., of
Mount Sinai Medical Center in New York City, who
has devoted many years to the search for better understanding of PMS, tells us: "A number of religions, which
remain with us today, viewed—and sometimes still
view—this very healthy and natural occurrence as
repugnant. When Moslem women are menstruating they
are not allowed to enter mosques. Women of Greek
Orthodox faith, early in this century, were forbidden
communion during their menstrual periods. At one time

in the Catholic church's history, intercourse during menstruation was a sin. Even though menstruation gives a woman a wondrous internal cleansing, in the Orthodox Jewish faith, a woman's 'clean' days are *after* her period, when she is immersed in a purifying bath."[1]

This feeling is not limited to any single ethnic or culture group; quite the opposite—researchers note that this same superstitious abhorrence exists throughout the world. Caroline Shreeve, M.D., a British physician, observes, for example, that "in a number of Australian tribes, a menstruating woman is severely scolded or beaten by her husband or nearest relative if she fails to warn approaching males of her condition.

"In other tribes of that continent the seclusion of menstruating women is even more rigid, and enforced by worse penalties than these—if, during her period, a woman of the Wakelbura tribe enters the encampment by the same route as the men, she may be put to death.

"The Bushmen of South Africa believe that a glance from a girl's eye at the time when she should be kept in strict retirement can fix men in whatever position they happen to occupy, with whatever they are holding in their hands, and change them into trees that are able to talk.

"Some societies dread the onset of female puberty even more than the recurrent menstrual flow. Among the Zulus and some other African peoples, the girls themselves believe that the sun shining on their heads during the arrival of their first period will wither them up into skeletons. This is why they hide away in the undergrowth with their blankets over their heads until the sun goes down, should the first signs of menstruation catch them unawares while they are working in the fields or gathering wood."[2]

During the early part of the twentieth century, the

same fears of the magical powers of menstruation persisted. Dr. Shreeve notes that in New Guinea, prepubertal girls were confined to tiny cages for four or five years before and after the onset of puberty; they were kept secluded in darkness and forbidden to set foot outside. When this confinement period ended, they were released to their marriage commitments.

Whether out of fear, ignorance or superstition, a menstruating woman has traditionally been ostracized or otherwise avoided. Simone de Beauvoir relates that in France, a menstruating woman is believed to have an adverse reaction on the curing of bacon, the fermentation of cider and the refining of sugar. In the Far East, menstruating women are not allowed to harvest the rice for fear that they might have a harmful effect on the crop. In South Africa, cattle is kept away from these women for fear that their presence might curdle the cows' milk.[3]

From the days of Hippocrates, healers have linked emotional crises to menstruation. "Women were flawed, not blessed, with this cycle of blood," says psychiatrist Ronald V. Norris, M.D., of the Premenstrual Syndrome Program, Inc., of Lynnfield, Massachusetts. "Some societies ensured a safe distance between menstruating women and others by banishing the women during their flow to special areas—tents, huts, a hillside—set aside for this purpose. This taboo was enforced to protect the group from damage to the crops and from the outbursts or behavior that were associated with menstruating women.

"Some of these cultures apparently thought there was a poison or 'menotoxin' in the menstrual blood. In part, this idea was inferred from the dramatic changes in bodily functions, attitude and behavior that some evinced each month just prior to the menstrual flow. As soon as the flow began, or within a few days of it, the woman's behavior would return to a normal state.

"Primitive peoples assumed that a toxic agent or spirit had caused the dramatic changes prior to menstruation and that once the menstrual flow began, the toxin was eliminated or washed away in the menstrual blood."[4]

Even in more recent times, this biological function has been shrouded in mystery and superstition. In any number of his lectures and writings, Sigmund Freud maintained that it was "penis envy" that created this emotional upheaval in women. According to Freudian theorists, women are envious of the male sex organ. Denied it, women go through episodes of "hysteria," temporary paralysis and a long list of psychosomatic ailments. Accordingly, males would keep a safe distance from such hysterical women, or confine them, which, no doubt, compounded the problem.

While this theory was satisfying to the Freudian group, it was not considered sensible by later psychologists, who relegated it to the category of superstition. One recent writer, Sheila MacLeod, who recounted her experience with PMS, says in *The Art of Starvation*, "I'm sorry to disappoint orthodox Freudians, but I felt NO penis envy, and I didn't think of myself to be maimed in any way . . . I was horrified and disgusted by menstruation rather than by sexuality. I felt that some dreadful punishment had been visited upon me, punishment for a crime which I had never committed. But I think I knew unconsciously that the supposed crime was twofold: I was being punished for being female and for having grown up."

Ms. MacLeod further comments that only girls, not boys, feel this sense of punishment during adolescence because "female changes traditionally were considered inappropriate for open discussion. *Boys'* development has always been treated as a mark of manhood."[5]

SYNDROME VS. TENSION

Throughout the nineteenth century, the process of menstruation gave rise to many strange notions. In 1878, the *British Medical Journal* debated whether menstruating women would cause food to become contaminated on contact. When this same journal was asked about providing medical education to females, the reply was: "If such bad results accrue curing dead meat while she is menstruating, what would result, under similar conditions, from her attempt to cure living flesh in her midwifery or surgical practice?"

Aside from the fear of blood, menstruation provoked another reaction that may have been responsible for the attitude that women were inferior because they could not control their bodies—namely, emotional tension. In fact, premenstrual syndrome was originally called premenstrual *tension*, because of the mental-physical outbursts that would frequently afflict women during their periods.

A pioneer researcher helped shed light on this condition. Robert T. Frank, M.D., of New York, methodically and carefully investigated the syndrome and referred to it as premenstrual tension in 1931. He prepared a paper, "The Hormonal Causes of Premenstrual Tension" and delivered it before a meeting of the Section of Neurology and Psychiatry at the New York Academy of Medicine. It set the stage for more understanding of this biological occurrence. He began his paper as follows:

"My attention has been increasingly directed toward a large group of women who are handicapped by premenstrual disturbances of manifold nature. It is well known that normal women suffer varying degrees of discomfort preceding the onset of menstruation. Employers of laborers take cognizance of this fact and make provisions for the temporary care of their employees. These minor disturbances include increased fatiguability, irritability, lack of concentration and attacks of pain.

"In another group of patients, symptoms complained of are of sufficient gravity to require rest in bed for one or two days. In this group, particularly, pain plays the predominant role. There is still another class of patients in whom grave systemic disorders manifest themselves predominantly during the premenstrual period."

Of this latter group, Dr. Frank reported that they "complain of unrest, irritability, 'like jumping out of their skin,' and a desire to find relief by foolish and ill-considered actions. Their personal suffering is intense and manifests itself in many reckless and sometimes reprehensible actions. Not only do they realize their own suffering, but they feel conscience-stricken toward their husband and family, knowing well that they are unbearable in their attitude and their actions.

"Within an hour or two after the onset of the menstrual flow, complete relief from both physical and mental tension occurs."[6]

Dr. Frank told of treating mild cases of this "tension" with diuretics; for those who had edema or excessive water, this was helpful. For the more severe cases, he used radiation to the ovaries. Dr. Frank's landmark paper opened the floodgates of research. It soon became apparent that the tension was only one part of the entire condition, hence a syndrome. But it did alert the public to the fact that emotional upset was a very real part of the condition.

It wasn't until 1947, however, that a pair of doctors, Harvey E. Billig, Jr., and S. Arthur Spaulding, Jr., were able to place the condition in its proper perspective. They found that many PMS symptoms could be eased with nutritional improvement, B-complex vitamins and correction of hypoglycemia (low blood surge swerve).

In an article in *Industrial Medicine*, they wrote that there was a "frequent striking clinical syndrome in women consisting of a triad of symptoms: a burst of energy several days before menses (premenstrual tension, easy bruising, and lowered threshold to pain). These patients, just prior to menses, feel the urge to do something such as cleaning the house, doing the laundry.

"They are hyper-irritable, crabby, and admit to being 'hard to live with.' Invariably, they will find black and blue marks on their bodies and often have no idea how they were incurred. Practically all of them are somewhat irritable and hyper-sensitive, and tend to flinch when someone touches them. There is usually a history of recurrent complaints of peripheral radicular [surrounding nerve] pains, which is usually the presenting complaint.

"They will readily admit that they 'just can't stand pain.' In many, considerable domestic difficulties are present, and frequently they are a serious problem. A fair percentage give a history of munching and nibbling between meals, and of increased nervous tension when meals are missed or delayed. Yet a surprising number eat little breakfast, and it is primarily the noon meal and the afternoon snacks which they rely upon 'to make them feel better.' . . ."[7]

Drs. Billig and Spaulding comment that glucose tolerance tests showed these women to be hypoglycemic just before onset of menstruation. This suggests that nutrition could ease the symptoms and control or even erase some of the often violent reactions of the condition.

It was not until 1953 that a well-known British physician, Katharina Dalton, herself subject to severe symptoms, decided to call the affliction premenstrual syndrome or PMS. In an article written with Raymond Greene in the *British Medical Journal*, she offered a better understanding of the condition and a call for a proper name:

"The term 'premenstrual tension' is unsatisfactory, for tension is only one of the many components of the syndrome. Its use has commonly led to a failure to recognize the disorder when tension is absent or is overshadowed by a more serious complaint.

"We have preferred to use the term 'premenstrual syndrome' but as our investigation has progressed it has become clear that this term also is unsatisfactory.

"Though the syndrome most commonly occurs in the premenstrual phase, similar symptoms occasionally occur at the time of ovulation, in the early part of the menstrual phase, and even rarely in the first day or two after the flow has ceased.

"The term 'menstrual syndrome,' though correct, for in each individual the symptoms recur at monthly intervals, may wrongly create the impression that they occur only at menstruation.

"We have finally decided to retain the term 'premenstrual syndrome' in the full realization of its imperfection. The full elucidation of its cause may later suggest a more appropriate and more accurate nomenclature."[8]

An official definition of the condition is given by the National Institute of Child Health and Human Development:

"Premenstrual syndrome (PMS) is the term given to the group of physical and behavioral changes that may affect some women in the week or so just before a menstrual period.

"For unexplained reasons, these women suffer moderate to severe distress and tension during that time. They may experience abdominal bloating, fatigue, irritability, or moodiness.

"Often they may do and say things that alienate friends and family. Negative self-images may develop as these women attempt to cope with severe symptoms."[9]

PMS OUTBURSTS IN FAMOUS VICTIMS

A number of celebrities in past and recent times displayed emotional outbursts of a periodic cyclical nature that have led endocrinologists to believe that PMS was to blame. Examples:

Queen Victoria. In her book *Once a Month*, Dr. Katharina Dalton decribes the emotional outbursts and temper tantrums of the eighteen-year-old Queen Victoria. She would hurl objects and scream at Prince Albert, her husband; she found fault with everything he did. Only when the queen was pregnant was she more rational. Observers noted that she would go into these tumultuous rages not only toward her husband but toward all around her in a cyclical pattern.[10]

Maria Callas. This brilliant opera singer was also known for her temperamental outbursts. Her biographer, Arianna Stassinopoulos, in a book entitled *Maria Callas*, tells of a pattern of such incidents. The negative outbursts, sinus attacks and binge eating (she zoomed to 250-plus pounds), plagued the diva from the end of the monthly cycle through the first ten days. In contrast, she was happy, serene and rational during the middle of the month.[11]

Judy Garland. The child star had no apparent difficulties during her early years, but apparently, when she approached puberty, she displayed irrational behavior which could be attributed to PMS. She, too, had temper tantrums, drunken bouts, trouble with whoever her husband was at the time, disagreements with her children. Her volatility, emotionalism, mood swings, depression and insomnia worsened after the birth of her

three children, according to biographer Christopher
Finch in *Rainbow*. She had mood swings and compul-
sive eating and weight problems; she became depen-
dent upon amphetamines and alcohol. It is possible that
the periodic problems were connected with PMS.[12]

Joan Crawford. Violent outbursts are described in
Mommie Dearest by the actress's stepdaughter, Chris-
tina Crawford. Miss Crawford was given to unprovoked
bouts of temper that terrified her stepdaughter. In the
biography, there are frequent references to the outbursts taking on a cyclic pattern.[13]

Mary Todd Lincoln. Wife of the president, she has
often been described as a woman given to emotional
outbursts, depression, migraine headaches. They were
most severe following the birth of her children. In his
biography, *Mrs. Abraham Lincoln*, author W. A. Evans
writes that Mrs. Lincoln was known for having hysterical outbursts. She is described as writing to a friend,
after Tad, her fourth child, was born in 1853: "I have
been seriously sick. (My disease is of a womanly nature,
which you will understand has been greatly accelerated
by the last three years of mental suffering.)" She is also
described as having sharp mood swings. "It was not
easy to understand why a lady who could be one day so
kindly, so considerate, so generous, so thoughtful and
so hopeful, could, upon another day, appear so un-
reasonable, so irritable, so despondent . . . and so prone
to see the dark, the wrong side of men and women and
events."[14]

Sylvia Plath. This famous poet, author of *The Bell Jar*
and other acclaimed works, was a victim of suicide. In
her own semi-biography, *The Journals of Sylvia Plath*,
she describes the sinusitis and mood swings that would
come and go on a monthly basis. She told of bad days
and good days. The end and beginning of each month

sent her down into the worst depression, suicidal thoughts, violent feelings. The middle of the month was bright. Granted, more detailed knowledge is needed before a final assessment can be reached. But based upon our new knowledge of the mood swings of premenstrual syndrome, we may well believe that Sylvia Plath's suicidal depression was due to hormonal upset.[15]

Chapter 2

DEFINING PMS

PMS is a multi-faceted reaction brought on by the cyclic activity of the hypothalamic-pituitary-ovarian network. It is characterized by many symptoms that recur regularly at the same phase of each menstrual cycle that is succeeded by a symptom-free phase in each cycle.

"Premenstrual syndrome (PMS) is a term for a number of symptoms and body changes that occur up to two weeks before each menstrual period," explains Brooks Ranney, M.D., of the American College of Obstetricians and Gynecologists. "Not all women are bothered by it, but many are to some degree. As many as 12 percent of all women of menstrual age, experts say, suffer symptoms discomforting enough to seek medical treatment, take time off from work or in some way disrupt their regular routine."[16] Among these symptoms, according to Dr. Ranney, are "nervous tension, irritability, fatigue, mood swings, mental confusion, general puffiness, bloating or swelling, weight gain due to retaining water in the tissues, breast tenderness, low abdominal ache, low backache and throbbing headaches."

Dr. Ranney explains that "precise causes are not known, but since the symptoms and findings recur with such regularity in some women, the causes appear to be related to the hormonal cycle." During the early part of each cycle, "ovaries produce the female hormone called estrogen. After ovulation, a second hormone, progesterone, is produced. This hormone is essential to maintain the health of any early pregnancy. It makes the lining of the uterus (endometrium) thicker, storing food and swelling the uterus. Also, it causes general body tissues to retain more sodium from salt which draws more water and fluid into body tissue spaces, causing swelling. Some premenstrual symptoms may be caused by this swelling in the uterus, pelvis, abdomen, legs, liver or brain," explains Dr. Ranney.

He also points out, however, that "although PMS is a real problem for some women, doctors involved in research on the subject caution against blaming it for all problems and ailments. Since many of the symptoms cannot be tested or measured, doctors suggest that if you suspect that you have PMS, you should keep a record during each menstrual cycle of what your symptoms are and when you experience them. This is the clearest way that you and your doctor can determine if you suffer from PMS."

Exact figures on how many women have the condition are hard to come by. Many women prefer to "suffer in silence" rather than seek help and are never identified in numbers. But we have a ballpark figure from James L. Breen, M.D., former president of the American College of Obstetricians and Gynecologists, who tells us: "One out of every five women between the ages of 25 and 40 may suffer from PMS that leave her temporarily disabled. These symptoms range from depression, aggression, irritability and anxiety to mood swings, nervous tension and food cravings. Physical symptoms include fluid retention, headache, acne, fatigue and exhaustion." He adds that while "most women can cope with *mild* forms of PMS, others with severe PMS, with physical and emotional stress, can be overwhelmed."

Some women (although a minority) have no symptoms of PMS and so are not included in any demographics. This is explained by Niels H. Lauersen, M.D., and Zoe R. Graves, Ph.D., of the department of obstetrics and gynecology at New York City's Mount Sinai School of Medicine.

"In a 1965 study, PMS was defined as any combination of emotional or physical features that occurred cyclically in females before menstruation, and which regressed or disappeared toward the end of menstruation.

"The investigators reported that, according to their definition, only 3 percent of their study group of healthy young women would escape being classified as suffering from PMS. Thus, it is important to distinguish between patients who describe premenstrual changes as tolerable or 'normal' and those who describe their symptoms as debilitating."

Drs. Lauersen and Graves list these symptoms: bloating, breast tenderness, irritability, tension, anxiety, depression, headaches, crying spells, increase in appetite, craving sweets, weight gain, pruritis, acne and joint pain. They agree that the exact incidence of premenstrual syndrome is difficult to determine. One investigator observed PMS symptoms in 40 percent of otherwise healthy women; another noted PMS in 36 percent of working women, and still another reported that 31.9 percent of 232 women with PMS had no organic disease that could explain their symptoms.[17]

According to the Medical and Pharmaceutical Information Bureau, Inc., "About 76 percent of women between the ages of fifteen and forty-four suffer from menstrual cramps, based on market research studies. Up to 90 percent of all women in their childbearing years experience at least some symptoms of PMS which may go beyond emotional manifestations such as irritability and depression, and include bloating and cramping among other symptoms."[18]

It is important to distinguish between PMS and dysmenorrhea, the medical term for painful menstruation. It is primarily caused by moderate to severe cramping of the uterus. Headache, backache, diarrhea and nausea are associated symptoms. The National Institutes of Health says, "In a recent health survey of adolescent women, more than half reported pain during menstruation."

Dysmenorrhea usually does not begin until six to twelve months following menarche (the start of the menstrual period, usually between the ages of ten and seventeen), when a woman's system has developed fully and ovulation occurs regularly. The disorder appears to affect young women and women who have *not* borne children more so than older women who have had children.

Medical specialists with the Upjohn Company in Kalamazoo, Michigan, explain, "Dysmenorrhea, or painful menstruation, affects about half of all adult women. Ten percent of them are believed to be incapacitated for at least several hours every month, many for a day or more.

"In economic terms, the best available data indicate that more than 140 million working hours are lost annually by the estimated 3.5 million American women who suffer severe dysmenorrhea. With the pain and lost time goes emotional distress."[19]

In other words, dysmenorrhea and PMS are responsible for more missed hours of work than colds or flu.

TWO THEORIES OF PMS

The exact cause of PMS is under scrutiny. At present, there are two basic schools of thought on the possible causes:

1. A hormonal imbalance stemming from disturbed rhythms or development in the hypothalamic-pituitary section of the brain—the brain's central switchboard and vital to the fulfillment of endocrine gland functions.

2. Excessive estrogen (female hormone) levels, inadequate progesterone (another hormone), a deficiency of vitamin B-complex and magnesium, disrupted glucose metabolism or hypoglycemia.

Whatever the cause, we know that PMS is real and not imagined. G. Timothy Johnson, M.D., of Harvard Medical School explains it this way: "Something happens physiologically in some women between the time of ovulation and the actual beginning of menstruation— the so-called luteal phase of the monthly cycle.

"During this time, women affected by PMS typically complain of a wide range of physical and emotional symptoms. Common emotional complaints are depression and anxiety, and physical symptoms include, among other things, fluid retention in the body, decrease in fine muscular coordination and fluid-filled breasts. It is important to stress that both the emotional and physical symptoms are cyclical: they occur only during part of the monthly cycle and are not persistent throughout the entire month, ending just before or during the very first few days of bleeding."

Dr. Johnson describes the popular theory that an imbalance in estrogen-progesterone hormone levels leads to the emotional-physical manifestations of PMS. But he adds that "there are no reliable laboratory methods of diagnosing this condition yet." Treatment, he concedes, is still a "hit or miss proposition. Most physicians sug-

gest beginning with a conservative therapy—a diet that
lowers the woman's intake of simple carbohydrates,
regular exercise programs and vitamin B6 (though there's
no proof of its effectiveness)."[20]

At least one out of every four women suffering from
severe PMS has attempted suicide or abused her husband or children, according to William R. Keye, Jr., of
the University of Utah Medical Center in Salt Lake
City. "I studied 89 women diagnosed as having severe
PMS. This is a disruption of normal personality and
other body processes."

Dr. Keye offers these startling discoveries:
  • 79 percent had seriously considered suicide; 12
    tried.
  • More than half suffered moderate or severe emo-
    tional stress.
  • 17 percent suffered other undiagnosed physical
    ailments.
  • 80 percent were helped with progesterone.

Dr. Keye felt that many women with severe symptoms could have violent reactions. "Even though these
women suffered severe effects prior to menstruation,
most functioned very well at other times."[21]

DO YOU HAVE PMS?

The pain and discomfort you feel once a month may
be due to PMS or to other causes. It is important to
know that PMS is a chameleon condition—it is frequently believed to be something else. And it is a
complex condition, too. No blood test can tell if you
have PMS (but it could identify the presence of another
disorder). Therefore, you should privately make an effort at self-diagnosis. First, you need to determine if
your symptoms are related to your menstrual cycle. If
so, you can find relief. Just keep a checklist and note if
you have regularly recurring symptoms just before your

period. The symptoms should occur *regularly*, precisely at this time. Such symptoms as headaches, nervousness, cramping, food cravings, crying urges or depression, either singly or with other symptoms, just before your period, could indicate PMS.

Also note if the *start* of your period brings relief from these symptoms. Again, this could indicate PMS. It would be a wise idea to have a general physical and/or gynecological checkup to rule out any organic cause for your symptoms. Cooperate with your doctor to diagnose PMS. Once it is identified, you can receive guidelines on how to cope with it.

SYMPTOMS AND CHARACTERISTICS OF PMS

PMS is characterized by a wide range of physical and emotional symptoms which occur at the same time of each menstrual cycle. The symptoms usually disappear when the cycle begins and recur only after a symptom-free phase following menstruation. No one woman will experience all the physical and emotional symptoms listed below; she usually has several of them.

Physical Symptoms

Feeling bloated	Change in bowel habits
Weight increase	Change in appetite
Breast pain/tenderness	Thirst
Skin disorders	Abdominal swelling
Hot flushes	Inflammation of the nose
Headache	Fluid retention
Pelvic pain	

Emotional Symptoms

Irritability	Insomnia
Aggression	Crying
Tension	Loss of concentration
Anxiety	Poor coordination/clumsiness
Depression	Mood swings
Lethargy	Confusion

Other characteristics of PMS include:

Adverse reaction to oral contraceptives (women with PMS usually tolerate the pill poorly);

Relief from symptoms during the last six months of pregnancy;

Development of toxemia during pregnancy;

Extended depression after childbirth;

Mistakenly attributing PMS symptoms to "early menopause";

Worsening of symptoms with age; and

Family history of women with similar symptoms, although without medical diagnosis of PMS.

Other facts about PMS:

An estimated 4 out of every 10 women suffer from PMS, to varying degrees, at some time in their lives.

Symptoms worsen with age. PMS may hardly be felt in the teen years; it is more common in the 20s and often serious by the mid-30s.

PMS afflicts women of all cultures, races and ages. For 10 percent of the sufferers, PMS is severe enough to cause serious disruption of their personal and professional lives.

PMS results in an annual loss of $10 billion to American industry because of absenteeism and lowered productivity.

PMS symptoms start anywhere from fourteen days to one day before menstruation; PMS is also characterized by a symptom-free period of a least one week after menstruation stops.

To be successful, treatment for PMS should be tailored to each individual woman. Treatment often includes a combination of diet and nutrition, emotional support, physical fitness and, when the symptoms are severe, hormone supplements. These methods will be discussed in detail further on in this book.

A word should be said about a condition called amenorrhea, which means loss of menstruation. It can be caused by upset hormones or may be traced to excessive physical activity such as jogging, cycling and strenuous dancing, as well as stress. Periods may stop because the constant exercise causes a weight loss and change in hormone balance.

While a woman experiencing amenorrhea is less likely to experience PMS, she is still susceptible to some of its symptoms. Her body is gathering estrogen because of a missed or halted period; this estrogen remains in the system and is not released through the normal flow. An estrogen overload can lead to headaches and other reactions.

If you have missed one or more periods, you would do well to have a checkup; with less physical activity or less emotional stress, your hormones will again be balanced and you will become regular again.

Chapter 3

HOPE AND HELP
FOR YOUR HORMONES

"HORMONES play an important role in the proper functioning of the menstrual cycle," according to the National Institutes of Health. And with a better understanding of how to control upset hormones, there is help for easing much of the misery of PMS.

The NIH offers this explanation of the entire menstrual process; note the heavy involvement of the endocrine system and the hormones it produces.

"The onset of menstruation (menarche) is the dramatic marker of the change from girl to woman. Usually occurring between ages of ten and sixteen, the beginning of menstruation means that a young girl is developing the ability to bear children.

"At first the cycle may be irregular. Usually, a regular menstrual cycle is established by the end of the first year after menarche. Interrupted only for pregnancies or specific health problems, it continues month after month until a woman is in her forties or fifties when menstruation ceases (menopause). A typical cycle is about 28 days, but cycles varying from 24 to 30 days are not uncommon. Generally, a woman keeps to the established pattern although stress, illness or the use of oral contraceptives may alter her cycle temporarily.

"During each cycle, the inner wall or lining (endometrium) of the uterus thickens to provide a suitable environment for a pregnancy. A mature egg (ovum) is released from one of the two ovaries in midcycle (ovulation) and remains in the reproductive tract for about three days. For a pregnancy to occur, the ovum must be fertilized by a sperm. If there is no pregnancy, the lining of the uterus breaks down and is discharged as the menstrual flow (menses) over the course of three to eight days.

"Although the reproductive organs are located in the body's pelvic area, the reproductive cycle is controlled by an area at the base of the brain containing the hypothalamus and the pituitary gland. The hypothalamus and the pituitary gland orchestrate menstrual cycle activities, sending 'start' and 'stop' signals each month to the ovaries and uterus.

"On the first day of menstruation, hormone levels are low. But after one week and for most of the remaining cycle, *estrogens* are produced to promote ovulation and stimulate the development of the endometrium. During this time, estrogens contribute to producing an appropriate environment in the reproductive organs for fertilization, implantation and nurturing of the early embryo. Estrogen production drops off a few days before the next cycle begins.

"*Progesterone*, a hormone produced in large amounts during the latter half of the cycle, stimulates the development of the endometrium in preparation for a pregnancy. If there is no pregnancy, progesterone levels decrease and menstruation begins. If pregnancy occurs, production of progesterone continues throughout the nine months to help maintain the pregnancy.

"Other hormone-like substances, *prostaglandins*, are also produced during the latter half of the cycle. Although the role of prostaglandins is not completely understood, they are believed to stimulate uterine contractions which are recognized as cramps during the menstrual period. The prostaglandins may be one of the possible factors that start labor."[22]

Medical research has confirmed that the cramps and other symptoms of PMS are caused by prostaglandins. If you experience more than "average" pain, you most likely have higher levels of this chemical in your body.

Because some of the prostaglandins escape into your bloodstream, they can affect other involuntary smooth muscles. That is one reason why some women suffer from backaches, nausea, diarrhea, dizziness, hot and cold flashes, fever and emotional tension, along with the painful cramping.

The NIH has also made a comprehensive study of the complex interrelationships of the hypothalamic, pituitary and ovarian functions. A new theory holds that certain messenger chemicals from the pituitary, neuropeptides, may be the cause of mood and behavior symptoms of PMS. The goal is to block action of these neuropeptides and thereby control the emotional reactions.

STRESS AND PMS

Basically, your brain's hypothalamus controls your menstrual cycle. This brain segment initiates the release of gonadotrophin (a follicle-stimulating hormone) which triggers the secretion of other brain hormones from the pituitary. Your cycle is under way. But there is a villain that can upset the rhythm. It is known as *stress*. It can disturb your delicate hypothalamus. It can upset your brain peptides (amino acid molecules) so that they cannot send normal nerve-transmitting signals that influence the working relationship between hypothalamus and pituitary.

After all, the brain signals that initiate hormonal fluctuations in the first place are susceptible to stress.
PMS, too, results from these hormonal fluctuations. If
you are under stress, there is an inhibition of hormone
release. You actually have a hormone deficiency that
can cause a severe imbalance, resulting in PMS.

PMS AND VIOLENCE

It was the noted British gynecologist Katharina Dalton,
herself a victim of PMS, who alerted the world to the
dangers involved in upset hormones. She reported that
49 percent of 156 women convicted of theft, soliciting
and drunkenness committed the crimes just before or
during menstruation. Of the 43 women (27 percent)
who complained of premenstrual symptoms, 63 percent
committed their offenses at the time of their symptoms.

Dr. Dalton commented that the tension accompanying PMS makes the woman helpless and puts her at the
mercy of her hormones; she cannot avoid violence,
especially with those closest to her.[23]

Ronald V. Norris, a Lynnfield, Massachusetts, psychiatrist who specializes in PMS, alerts us to the possibility
that "some violent acts committed by women may be
the result of a specially heightened mood." He tells of
studying aggressive behavior among women at a Massachusetts prison. "We interviewed six women who were
sentenced for murder—three victims were husbands,
two were children, one was a lover. Two things that
were striking about all six cases were that the killings
occurred on the day before or first day of menstruation,
and that all six women could have been described as
quiet, mild-mannered housewives."

According to Dr. Norris, "Outbursts of anger, the
throwing of objects, and on occasion even thoughts of
murder are fairly common in women with PMS. A

majority of women with PMS at some time or another, when under great stress or pain, say they have become angry, yelled, screamed, had a car accident, thrown something, or felt as if they wanted to throw something or act out against someone."[24]

Dr. Katharina Dalton has testified at numerous court cases involving women who committed violent crimes, including murder. In the *British Medical Journal*, she explained that PMS victims can be subject to violent moods. Furthermore, if a woman with PMS goes without food for long intervals, she can suffer hypoglycemia. This brings on a rush of adrenalin, a hormonal upheaval that can cause the woman to become enraged.

Dr. Dalton testified at the trial of an English girl who fell into a rage during a date with a young man. Before the night was over, she got into her car, drove right at the man and killed him. She was charged with murder using a deadly weapon (her car). Dr. Dalton said that PMS was one of a set of conditions to be considered. There had also been considerable drinking beforehand. This probably exacerbated the symptoms of PMS and the woman was hormonally driven to commit the murder.[25]

For many women, the symptoms of PMS can range from temperamental outbursts of short duration to more shocking violence that can snuff out the lives of others . . . or their own.

FOUR PMS GROUPS

Guy E. Abraham, M.D., of Rolling Hills Estate, California, has subdivided PMS into four major groups. Each one has specific symptoms, although there may be some overlap. This former UCLA professor, who specializes in PMS, has found that hormonal upheavals may be tamed with an initial identification of the specific group and nutritional guidance.

#1 PMS-A (Anxiety)

Symptoms: Chief complaints are nervous tension, anxiety, irritability and mood swings, occurring as early as two weeks before periods, becoming progressively worse, sometimes followed by mild to moderate depression and improving with onset of periods.

Cause: Elevated estrogens in the bloodstream. These ovarian estrogens stimulate the central nervous system to produce body stress. An ovarian hormone, progesterone, depresses the central nervous system for a calming effect. But during PMS, both hormones are produced in imbalanced quantities and this leads to PMS-A.

Treatment: Reduce intake of dairy products, refined sugar, animal fat. Boost intake of magnesium and vitamin B complex. Exercise outside once a day to ease tension.

#2 PMS-C (Cravings)

Symptoms: Increased appetite one to two weeks prior to onset of period. You have a binge-craving for chocolates or other sweets, especially when under stress. A few hours after indulging, you feel low and fatigued, with a pounding heart and headaches. You may have palpitations or the shakes.

Cause: Refined sugar triggers insulin release but in excess of your needs. These factors lower your blood sugar. Deficiency of a prostaglandin called PGE1 may also be involved. It suppresses insulin response to sugar and minimizes the nervous responses to decreased blood glucose.

Treatment: Cut down on animal fats. Use more vegetable oils; dietary cis-linoleic acid initiates release of PGE1. Unrefined, uncooked safflower oil is a prime source of cis-linoleic acid. Also boost intake of magnesium,

zinc, vitamins B3, B6 and C. Good magnesium sources
are whole grains, green leafy vegetables, legumes,
cereals.

#3 PMS-H (Hyperhydration)

Symptoms: Sensation of weight gain a few days preceding the period; swelling of the face, hands, feet.
Rings don't fit. Shoes become tight. Dresses are too
small in the waist. You feel bloated, with some congestion-
tenderness in lower abdomen and breasts. Often, weight
gain is less than three pounds but feels like much more.

Cause: Water retention. Elevated hormones of the
adrenal glands which control water and salt accumulation by the kidney. Brain hormones (ACTH) stimulate
these salt-retaining hormones. Excess refined carbohydrates increase brain serotonin to create this reaction.
Stress also activates the adrenal glands to release into
the bloodstream excessive amounts of salt-retaining hormones which potentiate the salt-absorbing effect of
insulin.

Treatment: Increased amounts of doctor-prescribed
vitamin B6 and magnesium; reduce salt-sugar intake.
Reduce animal fats. Increase use of vegetable oil. Vitamin E helps soothe breast pain.

#4 PMS-D (Depression)

Symptoms: Withdrawal reactions, depression, easy
crying jags, behavior or mood swings, contemplation of
suicide. Insomnia, forgetfulness, feelings of lethargy.
Difficulty in verbalizing.

Causes: Generally, forms of hypoglycemia; there are
low blood estrogens and contrasting high blood progesterone. Again, this indicates a hormonal upheaval.
Chronic lead poisoning causes depression. Lead blocks
the effect of estrogen on target tissues but does not

influence progesterone effect. Since progesterone is elevated during the last two weeks of the menstrual cycle, its depressing effect at that time is not counterbalanced by estrogen because lead blocks this estrogen effect. Chronic stress triggers adrenal hormones to upset endocrine balance in some susceptible individuals.

Treatment: It is important to test for lead toxicity and then help to remove this problem with proper diet. Adequate intake of magnesium will prevent lead poisoning by decreasing the absorption and increasing the excretion of lead. PMS-D requires proper medical care and should not be dealt with lightly.

Dr. Abraham feels that the "roller coaster" effect of PMS should be treated early to help both the sufferer and those close to her.

Easing the Symptoms

How can you ease PMS? The following general guidelines, based on modern findings from various medical sources, will help you cope.

1. *Determine If You Have PMS*. You may suspect you do but there is some uncertainty. You need to chart your symptoms. If you have this condition, then follow the rest of the program. Understand that you are not alone. The condition is biological, not psychological, and you can relieve symptoms with an adjustment in your lifestyle.

2. *Discuss PMS with Others*. Face up to it. You do need moral support. You need sympathy. You need the help of others—your husband, other family members, perhaps your employer. You can't always do it alone, so understanding from others is essential.

3. *Balance Your Blood Sugar*. PMS, for many, is a reaction accompanied by hypoglycemia. You can ease the symptoms by smaller and more frequent meals.

Reduce fat intake. Boost complex carbohydrates (fresh fruits, vegetables, whole grains). This helps ease distress throughout your cycle, especially after ovulation. You want to balance your blood sugar and a higher protein program is also helpful. Remember, when your hormone levels are changed, so is your biochemistry. You could be at high risk for nervousness, fear, sudden tearful outbursts, panic. Space meals at three to four hour intervals. No hunger pangs, please. A bedtime snack of salt-free cheese and crackers would be good.

4. *Regular Exercise and Fitness*. Plan for about thirty minutes on alternate days devoted to aerobic exercises. Bicycle riding (stationary, if indoors), swimming, fast walking, doctor-approved jogging are all good ways to elevate your mood and help sweep away the blues. Fitness is part of the program to ease PMS. It may well be the most important step.

5. *Omit Salt*. It absorbs water and this leads to bloating. Avoid adding salt when cooking and avoid high-sodium foods. Make fresh foods, instead of using very salty canned, frozen or processed foods. Use flavorful herbs and spices instead of salt.

6. *Have Bran Daily*. Your health store sells it; use it in wholegrain cereals, in blenderized beverages, in baking. Bran binds itself to water and facilitates elimination. Just two or three tablespoons of bran daily is important.

7. *Say "No" to Alcohol*. It can upset your hormone levels and worsen PMS.

8. *Vitamin Supplements Are Helpful*. While the whole group of B-complex vitamins is helpful, it is pyridoxine or B6 that is said to control bloating, help you resist depression and lessen your craving for sweets. A daily dosage of 50 mg with your doctor's approval should be helpful. Much more will be said about vitamins in the next chapter.

9. *Avoid Caffeine*. Pass up coffee, tea, cola and most soft drinks; chocolate, too. Check labels of patent medicines because many contain caffeine. Caffeine contains methylxanthines, substances which are believed to give rise to cysts in breasts. By reducing or omitting caffeine, you will find your breasts to be less sensitive during PMS. Switch to herbal teas, fresh fruits and vegetables and their juices to quench your thirst.

10. *Keep Calm . . . Cut Down on Stress*. Nervous tension can worsen PMS symptoms; remember, your glands are already on a collision course and under stress so you should be careful not to exacerbate the situation. Avoid tensions of any sort. Take time out to relax, nap, meditate, enjoy the outdoors. Less stress = less PMS.

11. *Enjoy Lovemaking*. For many women, a sexual climax will release bottled-up tension and this eases some of the discomfort of PMS. Your goal is to reduce pelvic congestion and one way is mutually satisfying lovemaking that culminates with your orgasm.

If you build this eleven-step program into your lifestyle, you should be able to ease PMS symptoms and enjoy life more.

Chapter 4
THE VITAMIN-MINERAL WAY
TO PMS RELIEF

NUTRIENTS may often be the missing link in your body's
health chain to correct the symptoms of premenstrual
syndrome. In some situations, just one nutrient can
balance your hormones and soothe your feelings. In
others, several nutrients and/or foods may be needed.
In either case, nutrition can play an important role in
your quest for relief of symptoms.

It was Dr. Morton S. Biskind who in 1943 first reported in the *Journal of Clinical Endocrinology and
Metabolism* that PMS symptoms were more painful in
women who had B-complex deficiencies. He suggested
treatment with rice bran extracts and brewer's yeast
and found that his patients showed much improvement.
These foods are prime sources of needed B-complex
vitamins.

In particular, Dr. Biskind reported that these vitamins were needed to stimulate the liver to deactivate
estrogen and thereby create a better balance in the
system. This discovery opened the door to the use of
nutrition as part of the treatment in helping to ease
PMS distress.[26]

In recent years, Guy E. Abraham, M.D., has also
reported that the "blues" of PMS can be relieved with

the use of appropriate vitamins and minerals. According to Dr. Abraham, "This field is going through a Renaissance period right now. New knowledge is rapidly accumulating to convince us that what we eat affects us in many ways. What I tell you today may have to be modified tomorrow. However, there are facts that cannot be denied.

"Our bodies evolved over thousands of years accustomed to a diet consisting predominantly of fresh fruits and vegetables, grains, nuts, legumes and cereals. Our endocrine system, the liver, the pancreas, the bowel have been accustomed to receiving complex carbohydrates which were slowly broken down into sugar and passed into circulation.

"The vitamins and minerals that help convert the food into energy and the building molecules of our body came together with the food. *Over the past century, we have gone away from this natural way. We are paying the price.*"[27]

How to overcome the PMS problem? Dr. Abraham suggests cooperation with your physician and a six-step basic program to help start you off:

1. Get closer to Nature. Avoid empty calories, junk food, soda pop, refined sugar and salt. Limit your intake of red meat.

2. Get adequate protein but not more than 1 gram per two pounds of body weight. The consumption of protein in the U.S. averages 100 grams a day. Too much protein pulls good minerals out of your body and increases further the demands for these minerals.

3. Magnesium helps calcium absorption and deposition in the bones where it belongs. Magnesium decreases the demand for calcium and calcium increases the demand for magnesium. Common sense then tells us to favor magnesium over calcium in our diet. In fact,

we evolved in an environment that was high in magnesium and poor in calcium, so our body developed a mechanism to conserve calcium. It does not have such a mechanism for magnesium.

4. Limit your intake of dairy products because they interfere with magnesium absorption, a mineral often deficient in American women. Dairy products have ten times more calcium than magnesium. You should favor foods that have at least twice as much magnesium as calcium.

5. Limit intake of coffee, tea, soft drinks and chocolate because they increase the demand for B-complex vitamins and may cause breast problems. Cut down on nicotine for the same reason.

6. Increase your intake of complex carbohydrates found in vegetables, legumes, cereals and whole grains. If you are not allergic to yeast products, brewer's yeast may be used as a flavor enhancer because of the high glutamic acid level. However, yeast is 7 percent nucleic acid and the maximum safe intake of nucleic acid per day is 2 grams. You should not take more than 2 tablespoons of yeast a day to be on the safe side, since you will be getting some nucleic acids from the other food you eat. Yeast is extremely rich in phosphate and you don't want too much of that either. Because of these limitations, you cannot get all your B-complex vitamins and trace element requirements from yeast alone.

A wholesome nutritional program helps balance the body's hormonal system, a key factor in easing distress. "One basic definitely bears repeating: The better your diet, the greater your energy, stamina, well-being and capacity to resist or overcome any bodily complaints— including those related to your monthly cycle," explains Patricia Allen, M.D., obstetrician/gynecologist and clinical instructor at the College of Physicians and Surgeons,

Columbia University of New York City, and co-author with Denise Fortino of *Cycles: Every Woman's Guide to Menstruation.*

"Along with a chronically stressful lifestyle, poor eating habits may contribute to menstrual distress—so keeping your nutritional house in order is essential to healthy menstruation."[28]

You can take the misery out of PMS with a corrective approach, improved nutrition, better understanding and the conviction that you can ameliorate your condition. Thanks to new knowledge available from nutritionists and physicians, we can clear up the misinformation about PMS and remove the sting from Eve's curse.

RELIEF FOR HEAVY BLEEDING

It is known that vitamin A levels in women do fluctuate in a regular pattern during the menstrual cycle. In one study, Drs. D. M. Lithgow and W. M. Politzer of Johannesburg, South Africa, tested the vitamin A levels in seventy-one women suffering from menorrhagia (profuse or prolonged menstrual bleeding) and found, on the average, only 67 international units (IU) of the vitamin per 100 milliliters of blood. By contrast, a group of healthy controls with normal menstrual periods had about 166 IU per 100 milliliters—almost two and one-half times the amount measured in the first group.

To make certain this was not a coincidence, the researchers then decided to treat fifty-two women with symptoms of dysfunctional bleeding with 60,000 IU of vitamin A each day for thirty-five days. Close to 93 percent of the women were either cured or helped by this treatment.[29]

BIOFLAVONOIDS

Heavy menstrual bleeding has also been shown to abate with bioflavonoids, according to a group of doctors at a French hospital who reported that these nutrients gave the women "good to excellent results."

Bioflavonoids, usually extracted for supplements from the inner peel and white pulpy portion of citrus fruits, are widely recognized in Europe for their ability to strengthen blood vessels, particularly the walls of the capillaries.

In treating menorrhagia with bioflavonoids, the French doctors observed "progressive improvement, with the most marked improvement achieved by the third menstrual cycle."[30]

VITAMINS AND OTHER SUPPLEMENTS

Vitamin E. R. S. London, M.D., a noted nutritional scientist at Sinai Hospital in Baltimore and Johns Hopkins University, believes that the symptoms of PMS can be alleviated with supplements. He and his colleagues gave a group of PMS volunteers either 150, 200 or 600 mg of vitamin E every day. A similar group of suffering women were given dummy pills in a double-blind test. Dr. London found that vitamin E, taken on a daily basis, helped to diminish PMS symptoms for most of the women. The response depended largely on the potency, with 300 mg being most effective. No side effects were reported.[31]

VITAMIN B6 (PYRIDOXINE)

This nutrient has been shown to be effective in relieving symptoms and preventing their recurrence. The over-the-counter drug panel at the Food and Drug Administration has reviewed this evidence, reaching the agreement that the vitamin is safe at "usual dosage levels." A good approach is to start with a small dose, around 50 mg, and await the results. If symptoms are not alleviated, gradual increases should be considered.

While vitamin B6 is safe at potencies around 300 mg, it is best not to go higher.

According to Leon Zussman, M.D., diplomate of the American Board of Gynecologists and Obstetricians, and affiliated with the Long Island Jewish-Hillside Medical Center of New York, "B-complex is essential to the health of the liver. And the liver plays a key role in neutralizing the excessive amounts of estrogen produced by the ovaries during the course of the normal menstrual cycle." Simply speaking, this suggests that the B-complex vitamins do offer protection against the hormonal upset of PMS.

This fact is emphasized by Texas physician John M. Ellis who has done extensive research on B6 and who thinks that it can relieve that heavy, bloated, puffy feeling so many women experience before menstruation.[32]

Barbara Seaman and Gideon Seaman, M.D., in their much acclaimed book *Women and the Crisis in Sex Hormones*, call attention to pyridoxine as being especially effective in alleviating the edema (fluid accumulation) that plagues the PMS victim. They write, "Some women with edema so severe that it cannot be controlled by potent diuretics (water pills) respond dramatically to B6 therapy. Pyridoxine can also produce speedy relief for breast engorgement and sometimes nausea and vomiting. Many women troubled with acne flareup before menstruation find that pyridoxine eases this reaction, too."[33]

A woman who has been taking a birth control pill over a period of time, but has now resumed normal menstruation, may have definite lapses in all bodily functions in which this nutrient plays an important role. The Pill may destroy pyridoxine almost completely. You need this vitamin for production of red blood cells and antibodies to fight disease; it also helps in normal function of the nervous system. The Pill may also destroy folic acid, a needed blood cell nutrient.

The Seamans suggest increases in protein—meat, fish, poultry, dairy products, eggs; lots of high-fiber foods such as bran, whole grains, seeds, nuts, peanuts, legumes and dark green leafy vegetables. They recommend vitamin C and bioflavonoids to correct a heavy menstrual flow, and they also suggest vitamin E, 200 milligrams, on a daily basis. This program, with exercise and a healthier attitude, should help ease symptoms, they say.

RELIEF REQUIRES MORE THAN ONE NUTRIENT

There is no scientific evidence to justify the use of any one single nutrient or substance for the treatment of premenstrual syndrome, says Joyce M. Vargyas, M.D., of the University of Southern California School of Medicine, Los Angeles. She calls for a wholistic or total body approach and individual programming.

Currently, standard therapy uses oral contraceptives, diuretics, progesterone and sedatives. But Dr. Vargyas would prefer to see PMS treated with nutrition "which is at least devoid of any serious side effects."[34]

A diagnosis should be based on the type and timing of the patient's symptoms, which should be present only during the luteal phase (the part of the cycle between ovulation and menstruation). "If the patient complains of problems throughout the cycle, the possibility of endogenous [from within] depression, anxiety neurosis or manic-depressive psychosis should be considered."

This approach is based on the theory that decreased dopamine (nerve transmitter) causes depression but increased or overload of estrogen causes anxiety. To help correct this imbalance, Dr. Vargyas recommends a high-protein diet "but low in salt and refined sugar. Vitamin B6 is prescribed particularly for anxious patients. The regimen also includes vitamin A for acne, vitamin E for breast tenderness and magnesium to decrease extracellular fluid [that which surrounds cells]."

One suggested etiology of PMS is ovarian steroid (hormone) abnormalities. Would administration of hormones be helpful? Dr. Vargyas feels that these results are contradictory. Some physicians find it is helpful; some find that the use of progesterone suppositories offers no clinical improvement. Dr. Vargyas prefers a total body approach, with the emphasis on nutrition.

If it has been medically confirmed that you have PMS, and not an underlying condition unrelated to menses, then you need to discuss nutrition with your clinician. This is the advice of Mona M. Shangold, M.D., of the Obstetrics/Gynecology Department at Cornell University Medical College. "Each patient requires adequate time for history taking in order to elicit an accurate picture of specific symptoms and their temporal relationship with menses.

"The women who experience premenstrual molimina [cycles] without significant inconvenience probably require no therapy. An explanation of cyclic hormone alterations is interesting and helpful to them. They usually glean an understanding and acceptance of their discomfort.

"Many of these women ask questions about these symptoms only because extensive PMS publicity has aroused their interest and concern. Many of them benefit from vitamin B6, pyridoxine, beginning with 50 milligrams a day throughout the cycle and increasing to 200 mg a day if symptoms persist."[35]

Drs. Guy Abraham and J. Hargrove treated women who had premenstrual anxiety with pyridoxine at the rate of 200 to 800 mg daily. They report that this therapy led to a decrease in serum estrogen, an increase in serum progesterone and an improvement in symptoms.[36]

Since pyridoxine is a cofactor required for catecholamine (nerve transmitter) synthesis, and since dopamine inhibits aldosterone (adrenal hormone) synthesis, note Drs. T. McKenna and D. Island, a deficiency in dopamine could lead to PMS depression and/or edema. The doctors suggest that pyridoxine administration could correct this catecholamine deficiency, thereby enhancing mood and alertness as well as reducing edema.[37]

Caution: You can get too much of a good thing, even from vitamins. Drs. H. Schaumburg and J. Kaplan caution that pyridoxine megavitaminosis (ingestion of 2000 mg or more daily) can lead to sensory neuropathy. The dosage should be physician prescribed.[38]

DRUGS VS. NUTRITION

Dr. Mona Shangold comments that a nutritional approach may be most helpful, in contrast to drugs. "Although Dr. Katharina Dalton has advocated the use of natural progesterone (200 to 400 mg by suppository) by PMS sufferers, reports of its success remain anecdotal and unproven by controlled study.

"Creation of a constant hormonal milieu by the use of a long-acting progestin has been reported informally to be successful in some cases. This effect may result from mere elimination of cyclic fluctuation in endogenous [internal] hormones."

Dr. Shangold adds, "Bromocriptine, a dopamine agonist, has also been used to treat PMS, with some success. While edema symptoms have responded well in these studies, placebos [dummy pills] also have been effective.

"Many women find premenstrual symptoms reduced when they exercise regularly and /or decrease salt ingestion. The role of exercise remains to be explained, while salt reduction probably decreases salt retention and consequent edema."

CHECKLIST OF IMPORTANT NUTRIENTS TO EASE PMS

The noted PMS specialist Niels H. Lauersen, M.D., author of *PMS And You*, advises an individualized nutritional program since each woman reacts differently to the monthly condition.[39] Hormonal balances do change from month to month, so specific potencies would be helpful. But Dr. Lauersen suggests a balance of nutrients to help prepare the body for the once-a-month occurrence and ease the syndrome. These include:

Calcium

About ten to fourteen days prior to menstruation, there is a drop in blood levels of calcium. This could cause muscle cramps, nervousness, abdominal/menstrual spasms, pelvic pain, bloating.

A PMS sufferer should take calcium but always together with magnesium since both minerals are bound in the body. *Caution*: Taking calcium alone can cause a magnesium deficiency.

Potency: The preferred form is calcium carbonate tablets, 500 mg each, with magnesium in doses of one-half that of calcium. Take one calcium carbonate tablet daily and two tablets during the fourteen days preceding the menstrual flow. For severe uterine cramping during the premenstruum, take one 500 mg calcium gluconate tablet with magnesium every two hours, but no more than six tablets a day. If this still does not ease pain, then take two tablets every two hours but do NOT go above six tablets a day.

Note: An oversupply of calcium will be passed off in wastes. But if you have kidney stones or any condition that calls for calcium monitoring, then discuss the dosage with your physician.

Magnesium

A deficiency of this mineral can cause PMS reactions such as muscle cramps, pelvic pain, nervousness and other symptoms similar to those of calcium deficiency. Remember, these two minerals work together to ease distress. If you increase magnesium, remember that it should always be one-half the calcium intake.

Potency: One 500 mg tablet of calcium carbonate each day should be taken along with 250 mg daily of magnesium. Increase your consumption to two daily calcium carbonate/magnesium tablets during the last half of your menstrual cycle.

"PMS and magnesium deficiency are involved in a vicious circle relationship," notes Guy E. Abraham, M.D. He tells of studying twenty-six PMS victims in the age group of twenty-four to forty-four. Together with his colleague, pathology professor Michael M. Lubran, M.D., he noted that all of these women had "significantly lower" red blood cell levels of magnesium than healthy controls.

Drs. Abraham and Lubran also note that stress, part of premenstrual syndrome, drains the body of magnesium. "Many PMS symptoms may be explained by a magnesium deficiency," they say. With the use of this mineral, together with calcium, the symptoms were relieved.[40]

Cramps are the leading cause of absenteeism among teenage girls in school, according to a 1981 survey based on National Center for Health Statistics data. As many as 14 percent of the teenage girls miss school because of menstrual cramps.

"That was certainly true of my daughter," says Bernard Horn, M.D., who practices in El Cerrito, California. "When she was sixteen or seventeen, she had such bad menstrual cramps that she would have to stay in bed sometimes for days." Dr. Horn gave his daughter codeine (a morphine-derived pain killer) but did not like using such a strong medicine. He recalled that magnesium was important in balancing female hormones and also acted as a natural diuretic.

He then gave his daughter 600 mg of magnesium daily when her cramps started. It worked like a charm. "That was thirteen years ago," says Dr. Horn, "and she has not been bothered by cramps since then."

Dr. Horn has seen this miracle mineral help ease PMS reactions for many women. "I usually suggest supplementing one of two ways. Most healthy people should take 400 mg a day, every day. This may help prevent discomfort during periods. But if a woman objects to taking the supplements every day, I tell her to do this: Starting five days *before* your period is due, take 600 mg daily and continue taking that amount every day until your period is over."[41]

Dr. Guy Abraham agrees, and he suggests that women take magnesium with vitamin B6 for better utilization. He tells of treating nine apparently healthy young women with a major flaw of having low blood levels of magnesium. "After the women took 100 mg supplements of vitamin B6 twice a day for four weeks, their blood levels of magnesium more than doubled! And in six out of the nine cases, normal levels were achieved."[42]

Zinc

An important mineral found in all cells and tissues, zinc is used to boost internal enzyme activity. It influences the DNA-RNA or genetic components of your body and this could have an effect on the severity of your symptoms. If you are zinc-deficient, your PMS symptoms may include irritability, depression, nervous upset and headaches.

Potency: Take 30 mg of zinc each day; boost to 50 mg immediately preceding your period. You may combine it with calcium and magnesium. *Caution*: Do not take zinc with iron as these minerals are antagonists and block each other's absorption into the bloodstream.

Stress, notes Dr. Abraham, is a part of PMS, and it is zinc that is able to ease cramps and other symptoms. "Zinc is very good at clearing up skin problems and cramps, too. *Reason*: zinc regulates the body's production of prostaglandins, those hormone-like substances that bring on uterine contractions and cramps. Zinc is able to help control prostaglandin overload and protect against cramps."

Vitamin E, too, according to Dr. Abraham, is helpful. It increases circulation and thereby increases the amount of blood carrying oxygen to the uterus. Thus, when the uterus contracts, more blood and oxygen can pass through. When there is a restriction of this blood-to-oxygen-to uterus route, then cramps occur. Vitamin E helps reduce the pain that results.

Iron

A most essential mineral because it protects against anemia, fatigue and weakness. Because of iron loss many PMS sufferers become extremely tired to the point of depression. This could be corrected with adequate iron in the system. Also note that a woman who loses a lot of blood during her period is at high risk for an iron deficiency.

Potency: Take 30 mg three times a day, every day of the month; the preferred form of iron is ferro-gluconate or ferro-sulphate. You could also try one long-acting iron capsule each day. For better absorption of iron, take vitamins C and E at the same time. *Example*: The 30 mg of iron (three times a day, remember) should be combined with 1000 mg of vitamin C and 200 IU of E. *Note*: If you still have the symptoms, you could be anemic because iron and/or vitamin B12 cannot be absorbed properly. You need to consult your health specialist.

Potassium

This mineral is considered an electrolyte, that is, a solution that produces ions. An ion is an atom or group of atoms that conduct electricity. Electrolytes are needed to help your body fulfill needed obligations. For example, potassium influences levels of fluid retention; if you feel waterlogged, you could be deficient in this essential electrolyte.

Caution: Taking diuretics and/or improper diet may be the reason for the deficiency. This causes sodium and fluid buildup in your body cells. Symptoms include chronic tiredness, weakness and headaches. You may also have difficulties in the cardiovascular and muscular systems because potassium involves these responses, too.

Potency: Two tablets, four times daily, after meals and at bedtime, with potency of 5 milli-equivalents (mEq.) of potassium gluconate per tablet. This will give you a total of 40 mEq. of potassium. If you have severe PMS, then you may need two or three times this amount; for a healthy woman, any surplus is given off in wastes. If you have renal (kidney) or cardiovascular problems, then get your doctor's okay before taking this mineral. For these conditions, an excess can cause irregular heartbeat and potential fatality if a renal condition exists, too. (Potassium may irritate the gastrointestinal system for some; it may predispose to ulcers. Check your reactions and discuss its use with your physician.)

Health stores have potassium in doses of either 83.5 or 99 milligram tablets. This dosage equals about 5 mEq. of potassium gluconate. It's important to check labels.

Vitamin A

Needed for building up your immune system and helping your body fight off infection, illness and symptoms such as those of PMS. Since PMS can weaken your resistance, especially if you are under any type of stress, this vitamin is most helpful.

Potency: Take 5000 units, three times a day, together with your other vitamins.

Vitamin B Complex

Very much needed by the average woman. A typical diet will be deficient in this group, because it is water-soluble and easily lost during processing or cooking. Whole grains that are stored for a period of time or exposed to light also lose this perishable nutrient.

Vitamin B complex is needed to help your body regulate production of estrogen; a deficiency could cause an endocrine imbalance and as estrogen overloads, there is intense pain during menstruation.

Vitamin B6 or pyridoxine is the B-family member you need most. It influences the release of dopamine and serotonin, two brain neurotransmitters that help regulate your mood. A pyridoxine deficiency means a dopamine-serotonin deficiency, making the PMS victim feel tense, depressed, nervous, easily agitated. There may be increased eating urges and accumulation of fluid.

For relief, you need to take pyridoxine but ONLY in combination with the rest of the B-complex family to maintain a balance. This is important! You want to have accurate and steady neurotransmitters and this can be done only with a proper balance.

Potency: Take 100 mg of vitamin B complex together with 50-200 milligrams of B6 throughout the month. Two weeks before your period, boost potency of B6 to 500-800 mg daily. But remember, taking it alone can be risky and also cause stomach upset so include it with the rest of the B complex. This combination is said to be the most effective in easing distress, often eliminating most symptoms.

Vitamin C

Important for constructing collagen, the cement-like substance of connective tissue that maintains health of the body cells. It also strengthens your capillaries, builds iron in your bloodstream and protects against oxygenation of other essential nutrients. Since PMS causes destructive stress, it is important to have it in your system daily. Remember, it is water-soluble, easily destroyed and not stored by your body.

Potency: At least 2000 mg of vitamin C each day.

Vitamin D

An important vitamin that is produced on your skin when you are in sunlight. If you spend much time indoors, you could be deficient in this nutrient. It is needed to build calcium into your body. Since it aids in calcium absorption, take it together with calcium and magnesium supplements.

Potency: Aim for 400 units of vitamin D once a day, to boost the effectiveness of calcium and magnesium in easing your symptoms. *Caution*: A vitamin D deficiency means discomfort and pain!

Vitamin E

There is considerable debate over the effectiveness of this nutrient in easing PMS. Some studies show that taking 400 or more units of vitamin E daily for upwards of three months improves fibrocystic breast disease (also caused by hormonal imbalance). Other studies show that it does not help. But there is no denying that this is an important nutrient. It helps to protect against the oxidation of fatty substances such as vitamin A and essential fatty acids, as well as adrenal, pituitary and sex hormones. It has a protective action which helps establish good hormonal balance.

Potency: Between 400 and 800 units daily.

Dr. Niels H. Lauersen comments, "The natural approach, which includes a nutrition program, mineral and vitamin supplementation, and methods of stress reduction, is the first line of treatment for PMS. A woman may plan her own natural approach after she identifies her PMS symptoms."[43] And of course it is important to be under the care of a PMS doctor.

Chapter 5
YOUR PMS DIET PROGRAM: THE HYPOGLYCEMIA CONNECTION

MANY PMS SUFFERERS are addicted to processed and fast foods and sugar in just about any form. This gives rise to the problem known as hypoglycemia, or low blood sugar. It affects close to 40 million Americans, more women than men, especially women between the ages of thirty and forty. And it can be disastrous during PMS.

True, there are many women who have hypoglycemia but are free of PMS. But many women do have altered glucose tolerance levels during the luteal phase, or last half, of the menstrual cycle. There is a connection. It needs to be identified and then cleared up.

Hypoglycemia means low blood sugar, or a condition of faulty glucose metabolism in which an increased outpouring of insulin actually drains the body of glucose. (All sugars taken into your system are changed into glucose or blood sugar.) Since every single body cell needs glucose to function, if you have "glucose starvation," your entire body begins to react.

Why do you have such unusual carbohydrate or sugar cravings during PMS? It could be a manifestation of hypoglycemia. During the luteal phase, your cells bind insulin and create a high insulin level in your body. A high insulin level causes your blood sugar to fall much more speedily. If you are in the midst of PMS and bothered by the urge to eat sweets, you most likely have a high insulin-low blood sugar imbalance. If you surrender to the urge to eat concentrated sugar, you could bring on a hypoglycemic attack. Instantly, the sugar pours into your bloodstream. Your too-high insulin goes even higher, and this causes your low blood sugar to go lower. This can happen within half an hour after you eat sweets and may bring about a worsening of symptoms.

Health-science writer Jane Brody of the *New York Times* explains it this way: "Insulin overshoot, as doctors call the overproduction of insulin in response to a sugar load, happens to some extent to everyone who consumes a concentrated dose of sugar, especially between meals.

"It's probably an evolutionary hangover from our early days as a species when the only sources of sugar in the human diets were fruits and vegetables, which come into the body diluted by other digestible nutrients plus water and fiber. The body was not designed to handle sugar in concentrated forms, such as a piece of cake or candy bar."[44]

Biologically, most body cells are able to store some amounts of glucose—but not your brain! It must have a steady glucose supply from your bloodstream. If deprived of glucose, your brain becomes exhausted. It malfunctions.

It is your hypothalamus that controls glucose regulation. When your body nerve receptors signal your hypothalamus that hypoglycemia exists, there is a speedy reaction. Immediately, there is a reduction in the amount of glucose otherwise destined for your brain and peripheral cells, especially your muscles. This sudden imbalance of glucose triggers hypoglycemic-like symptoms, including weakness, tremulousness, constant hunger, sweating, throat constriction, anxiety, nervousness, irritability and accelerated pulsebeat. This set of reactions persists, even worsens, until you have fresh glucose from food or from storage-depots in your liver to nourish your brain.

PMS + HYPOGLYCEMIA

While many women have one without the other, most have PMS because they have hypoglycemia concurrently. During this once-a-month upheaval, there are changes in glucose tolerance, and even if you have normal glucose blood levels, your body is so sensitive, there is still a hypoglycemic-like reaction. It is estimated that one out of every ten women has this combination. Even if you do not have diagnosed hypoglycemia, you may have these symptoms because you have a reduced threshold for glucose during your symptomatic phase, which triggers off the distress of body and mind.

To determine if you have hypoglycemia, you will need to have a glucose tolerance test which tabulates the rate of sugar metabolism in your body over several others; this is done after fasting and then ingesting a supervised amount of carbohydrates and sugars. A diagnosis may show a flattened glucose tolerance curve which means you have an increased tolerance for sugar, not altogether desirable for your condition. Once hypoglycemia is diagnosed, dietary treatments can be outlined.

YOUR PMS DIET PLAN

Perhaps the most important rule of this plan is to avoid refined sugar. Refined sugar will trigger the release of an excess of insulin. A few days prior to the onset of your period, your body is very insulin-sensitive; refined sugar can be devastating. You could experience the emotional-physical effects of plunging blood sugar levels. This will worsen the effects of PMS on your general health, as well.

Basic rule: Say "no" to anything that contains refined sugar. Remember, it is the fastest of all foods to be absorbed into your bloodstream and this can cause severe reactions. No sugar means less PMS, because of decreased risk of hypoglycemia. Then follow these guidelines:

1. Eat several small meals throughout the day instead of the two or three basic large ones; plan for six such meals. Have main ones, but also have a mid-morning, mid-afternoon and pre-bedtime snack. It helps stabilize your digestive system.

2. If you are not on a diet, then aim for about 1500-2000 calories per day. To lose weight, consult your physician for guidelines.

3. Plan for a maximum of three ounces of red meat each day. Your protein count should be 4 ounces daily for 1000 calories, 6 ounces daily for 1500 calories, 12 ounces daily for 3000 calories. (Make protein from 15 to 20 percent of total daily calorie intake.) Select from: very lean meats, fish, poultry, whole grains, beans, meat substitutes or analogs. Limit dairy products (eggs, milk, yogurt, butter, cheese) to two small servings a day.

4. Boost intake of complex carbohydrates (whole grains, seeds, nuts, vegetables, fruits), which are metabolized into needed glucose but at a slow rate. *Note*: Proteins and fats are very slowly metabolized to give a persistent and gradual rise in blood sugar to ease distress.

5. Be moderate in intake of fats; plan for less than 20 percent of calories a day from polyunsaturated fats

(vegetable oils). These, too, give you a gradual rise in blood sugar.

6. Say "no" to salt. It leads to fluid retention (edema) and bloating. The swelling is noticeable several days prior to onset of menstruation. *Caution*: There is salt in soft drinks, tonics, club sodas, many packaged desserts. And salt is part of almost *all* processed, frozen, canned and bottled foods and beverages. Read labels. It is best to prepare your own foods to avoid salt. Try salt-free mineral water, seltzer, tap water.

7. Reduce or eliminate caffeine, too. It is found in coffee, chocolate, tea, most soft drinks (check labels). Caffeine acts on the receptor cells for adenosine, a natural body substance that has an affinity with caffeine and influences many physiological processes that require energy. You may have a boost in energy, but a letdown as your blood sugar goes through a "yo-yo" reaction. Switch to caffeine-free products.

8. Boost your consumption of wholegrain products, green leafy vegetables, legumes.

9. An exceptionally good food is safflower oil; it is a prime source of cis-linoleic acid, a predecessor of prostaglandin El, which can buffer symptoms of PMS.

10. Never skip meals. Eat as slowly and leisurely as possible. You will help fuel your body with a steady and balanced food supply so you have glucose at a regular level.

Whether you have diagnosed hypoglycemia or just a "lowered glucose tolerance" or sensitivity to sugar, you will have insatiable urges to eat, even when you're full. The reason is that excess refined carbohydrates boost brain release of serotonin, which in turn provokes the eating urge that then brings on weight gain. It is all part of the sugar-triggered insulin outpouring. With the preceding ten-step rule (and, most important of all, the elimination of anything containing sugar), you should help balance your blood sugar and control the urge to overeat.

Tip: Try a bit of protein with a carbohydrate. The reason is that protein needs more time to enter your bloodstream and become glucose; in contrast, carbohydrates enter your bloodstream very rapidly, making a demand for insulin to convert the glucose. More insulin may cause a blood sugar drop and this sets off a PMS mood reaction. *Suggestion*: Eat an orange, pear or apple with a piece of cheese. You have your protein-carbohydrate pair and this moderates insulin production and balances blood sugar.

FOOD PLUSES AND MINUSES DURING PREMENSTRUAL PHASE

The goal is to balance hormonal levels. You can do this with these healthful foods:

Fruit juices (especially orange or grapefruit juice, although these should be kept to a minimum because of the high concentration of natural sugar); all fresh fruits, especially potassium-rich bananas; fresh vegetables, and their juices; frozen or canned vegetables but ONLY if salt and sugar free. Yogurt, if sugar free; eggs; cheeses free of salt and sugar; hot or cold cereals without salt; salt-free wholegrain breads; wholegrain pasta products; brown rice; fresh but lean meats, fish and poultry; nuts and seeds without salt; popcorn without salt or fats; butter without salt; moderate amounts of honey or jams, but without added sugar.

Since PMS has been directly connected to fluid retention because of salt, especially during the luteal stage of your cycle, you need to say "no" to this seasoning in any form. No salt from the shaker. No salt in cooking. And avoid these, too: Potato chips, pretzels; buttermilk and cheese (except if labelled salt free); processed meats (canned, pickled, dried or smoked).

Avoid canned vegetables and juices unless salt free; salted butter and margarine; peanut butter, packaged breads and cereals. Canned soups, whether ready-to-eat, dehydrated, powdered, bouillon cube, etc., are also high in salt. Commercial soft drinks and prepared desserts, salad dressings, soy sauce, catsup, relish, horseradish, olives and gravies are all high in salt. Say "no" to anything that contains MSG (monosodium glutamate).

Tip: Because most restaurant foods, fast or otherwise, are high in salt (and sugar, too), unless specified, you would do well to eat at home during your premenstruum. You'll be much safer and have balanced blood sugar, too.

SAMPLE MENU PLAN FOR
BEATING THE PMS BLUES

Use this as a guide with appropriate substitutions. Again, remember to remain within your caloric limits and, when using alternative items, the "no salt, no sugar" rules still apply.

Breakfast

A citrus fruit half; a soft-cooked egg; a platter of fruit and cheese; low-fat cottage cheese or yogurt; wholegrain toast.

Important: It is best to avoid fruit juice in the morning; it has a high concentration of sugar which could cause an insulin overpouring and reduction in blood sugar, which are not advisable first thing in the morning.

Lunch

Vegetable-sprout salad; add diced chicken or turkey, or tuna; enjoy cucumbers, tomatoes, lettuce or seasonal vegetables.

Make a dressing of tomato juice, lemon juice, diced garlic. You could use safflower oil whch is a prime source of the needed linoleic acid. *Caution*: oil is calorie-high, so if you are trying to lose or control weight, use in moderation; one to two teaspoons should be sufficient.

Dinner

Baked potato; lean meat, fish or poultry; have a hot or cold vegetable salad. Try alfalfa sprouts, asparagus and green leafy vegetables, all of which are said to be natural diuretics. Fresh fruit for dessert.

Between-Meal Snacks

Peanut butter/banana sandwich on wholegrain bread; fruit/cheese combo; meat substitute slices/greens; yogurt/cheese. (These are typical carbohydrate-protein combinations that help keep your blood sugar steady. Plan to eat at three-hour intervals.)

Try tahini (sesame seed-butter) on wholegrain bread or tofu (soy cheese) with fruit slices. Enjoy cottage cheese and fruit sprinkled with wheat germ.

Other good snacks: apple, orange, grapefruit; melba toast; salt-free pretzels, popcorn (no butter), zwieback toast, wholegrain crackers, graham crackers, angel food cake without icing, assorted nuts, seeds (without added fats or salt). Almost any fruits that are fresh; if frozen or canned, the label must say there is no sugar added. Quench your thirst with fruit juices; homemade are best. If frozen or packaged, read label to determine if sugar has been added. If in doubt, pass it up.

NATURAL TONIC FOR PMS RELIEF

Start the day off by boosting your blood sugar and balancing your insulin levels with a highly nutritious blenderized tonic. It is a rich concentration of the valuable B-complex vitamins, protein, calcium, magnesium, vitamin E and other nutrients that ease PMS.

Combine one-half cup of sugar-free plain yogurt, 1 tablespoon brewer's yeast, 1 tablespoon bran, 1 tablespoon wheat germ, 1 banana, ½ cup of skim milk. Whirl in your blender for 30 to 60 seconds. Drink slowly.

Try this natural tonic as a breakfast and see if it helps you experience more freedom from symptoms.

Niels H. Lauersen, M.D., and Zoe R. Graves, Ph.D., of Mount Sinai School of Medicine in New York, also suggest the use of a natural approach in easing the symptoms of PMS.

"A 'natural' approach in counseling may be combined with medical treatment. Initially, the patient is advised to decrease her caloric intake. Increased body weight and the conversion of fatty tissue to estrogen may exacerbate PMS symptoms.

"Patients are encouraged to increase physical activity and exercise in order to promote metabolism and rebuild muscle mass.

"A low-salt diet will help avert premenstrual water retention and edema.

"Many patients also seem to benefit from low-sugar intake; some have even been encouraged to remain on a hypoglycemic diet, since the reduction in blood sugar fluctuation often has been found to have a positive effect on the elimination of PMS symptoms."[45]

The noticeable symptoms involved in the premenstrual cycle may be Nature's signal that your body requires extra care and dietary help during this trying time. Be alert to your physical needs. Nourish yourself. Learn sensible eating habits. You will help increase your chances of coping successfully with PMS . . . even eliminating it!

Chapter 6

PROGESTERONE—
THE KEY TO PMS CONTROL?

DURING THE 1930s, several scientific research teams announced the discovery of *progesterone*, one of the major sex hormones secreted by women throughout their reproductive lives.

Produced by the ovaries, the adrenal glands, and by the placenta in pregnant women, progesterone prepares the uterus for the reception and development of the fertilized egg and causes enlargement of the breasts during pregnancy and after childbirth.

Since its discovery, this hormone has been so closely linked to PMS that it has been suggested and prescribed as a means of keeping the symptoms under control.

Countless women (and the men who live with them) have become so eager for a "cure" that they eagerly look to this hormone as a magic bullet. And in clinical studies, it has been found helpful in the sense that it eases symptoms and reduces the severity of PMS. But remember that the menstrual cycle is still under scrutiny by scientists and many kinds of medication are being investigated.

To better understand what progesterone can and cannot do, you need to know what some of the key words mean.

Progesterone. One of the two major female sex hormones. It is produced by the ovaries and adrenal glands, and by the placenta in pregnant women. *Natural* progesterone prepares the uterus for the reception and development of the fertilized egg. *Synthetic* forms of progesterone—used in oral contraceptives—inhibit ovulation. Pharmacists have created a molecularly identical compound in synthetic form that may be used as an injection or suppository for the relief of PMS symptoms.

Progestin. Any natural or synthetic substance whose activity in the female body is similar to that of the ovarian hormone progesterone. It is a generic term; it is used interchangeably with progestogen.

Progestogen. A female hormone similar to progesterone; it is one of a group of naturally occurring or synthetic steroid hormones, including progesterone, that maintain the normal course of pregnancy. Progestogens are used to treat PMS; because they prevent ovulation, they are a major constituent of oral contraceptives.

Steroid hormones. Substances derived from cholesterol; they consist of three six-membered carbon rings and one five-membered carbon ring. Naturally occurring steroids include the female hormone estrogen, the hormones of the adrenal cortex, progesterone, bile salts and sterols. Synthetic steroids have been produced for therapeutic purposes.

Over the years, many scientists theorized that if the basic cause of PMS could be pinpointed, a possible cure could then be suggested. One possible cause was thought to be a decline in body production of progesterone. If the deficiency could be corrected, PMS symptoms could be relieved.

Progesterone was first isolated by Willard Allen, M.D., in 1934 and it was used successfully for easing symptoms of PMS. According to his published reports, it helped many women. It also opened the door to further understanding of the syndrome.

A possible cause of PMS was identified by Leon Israel, M.D., in 1938, as being an uncontrolled estrogen reaction traced to a deficiency of progesterone. Dr. Israel subsequently documented studies of the luteal phase steroid levels (the part of the cycle *between* ovulation and menstruation is referred to as the luteal phase) to show that the estrogen-progesterone imbalance was the problem. For millions of women, correcting the imbalance appeared to be a solution.

But there are conflicting views on just what does cause PMS. Dr. Ronald V. Norris of Tufts University says that the syndrome may actually be several diseases. "If progesterone works, it may be because some cases of PMS are due to progesterone deficiency, and others relate to some abnormality in the hypothalamus-pituitary axis on which progesterone has some effect."[46]

Dr. Katharina Dalton of the University College Hospital in London, one of the pioneers of PMS and founder of London's Premenstrual Syndrome Clinic, has repeatedly stated in many medical journals that the symptoms are caused by a deficiency of progesterone in the last phase of the menstrual cycle. She claims to have achieved a 95 percent cure rate by treating patients with natural progesterone in the form of injections or suppositories.[47] (Natural progesterone is different from progestogen, the chemical hormone used in birth control pills that has been associated with blood clots and other reactions.) Her procedure is under scientific scrutiny and has received praise as well as criticism.

Dr. Dalton alerted the world to the possibility of solving the hormonal riddle of PMS with something as simple as progesterone. In her book *Once a Month* she offers endless case histories of women who were troubled with reactions from the benign to the bizarre and were rescued from the torment of PMS with the use of progesterone supplements.

Dr. Dalton's rule of thumb is that progesterone needs to be administered in potencies higher than the amount the average woman produces herself during a normal menstrual cycle. These hormonal megadoses are considered safe, according to Dr. Dalton.

Progesterone is made from yams and soybean plants. It cannot be taken in pill form because, being a natural hormone, it is speedily broken down by the digestive system and eliminated from the body before it can do its work.

It is available as a prescribed treatment in any of these forms:

Injections. These are said to be painful, with such side effects as dizzy spells, amenorrhea, delayed or early menses, increase or decrease of the flow, weight fluctuation, change in sex drive. Because it creates a euphoric feeling, it could be addictive.

Vaginal Suppository. These are leaky; sometimes they can cause vaginal or rectal burning and irritation. The powder gives off a gritty-bitter reaction; the fluid has to be inserted with a basting syringe, not very comfortable, to say the least.

Liquid Insert. When introduced into the vagina, it has an irritating reaction.

Powder Insert. This may be placed beneath the tongue or in the rectum; in either situation, it is uncomfortable and may produce nausea.

Suppository Potency. Basically, the woman starts with a 200 milligram dosage each day throughout the premenstrual phase. (This contrasts with the 0.3 milligram to 2 milligram dosage in most birth control pills.) If the symptoms are not eased, then megadoses from 400 to 1600 milligrams daily are taken.

The use of progesterone is still a subject of controversy and is a highly individual matter to be discussed by each patient and her physician.

"The Food and Drug Administration has not approved large-scale manufacture of the drug, but physicians are not prohibited from prescribing it. There is data linking progesterone to cancer in laboratory animals," cautions *Science News*. "The major evidence supporting progesterone therapy comes from Dr. Katharina Dalton who has been treating PMS patients with the drug for years; she estimates that if PMS is carefully diagnosed, about 80 percent of the patients should respond to progesterone. She has never done systematic, controlled studies, however."[48]

Mention is also made of the reason for the confusion. Dr. Jean Endicott, a psychologist with Columbia University, explains that all of the existing studies have mixed together subjects with a wide range of symptoms and called them all PMS. "There is no one premenstrual syndrome," says Dr. Endicott. "Some women are anxious and agitated. Some are angry. Some are lethargic and overeat, while others have insomnia and don't eat. It's highly unlikely that the same biological variables are involved in hypersomnia and insomnia."

There are different types of PMS, some more extreme than others, which would make it difficult to prescribe one so-called cure (progesterone) for all.

The suppository form of progesterone appears to be best tolerated by most women. Pharmacists are permitted to compound suppositories for individuals with a physician's prescription. But in order for a pharmaceutical manufacturer to make them *en masse*, more research must be completed and approved by the FDA before permission is granted.

Dr. Katharina Dalton insists there is safety in the megadoses of the hormone. "It is impossible to give an overdose of progesterone to a woman who has borne children, because during pregnancy women are exposed to a fifteenfold increase in their blood progesterone levels for nine full months, instead of just a mere two weeks, and the body has learned to deal with that," she says.

What of women who have not given birth? Dr. Dalton concedes that with megadoses of progesterone, they may occasionally experience menstrual cramps, feel euphoric, show nervous energy and have bouts of insomnia. But she labels these as *"minor* side effects." Again, since each woman is different, what is minor to one may be major or disastrous to another.

THE NEGATIVE SIDE OF PROGESTERONE

Proponents say that progesterone is a natural hormone that takes up the deficiency in the body that is believed to be responsible for symptoms. But is a progesterone suppository a natural supplement? Many physicians will say that this supplement has the same properties as the progesterone made by the body, and therefore may be considered natural.

Fact: The ONLY natural progesterone is that which is made in the body!

Fact: The "natural" product given to you via a prescription at your pharmacy has been manufactured in a laboratory. It is *synthetic*!

Fact: The prescribed suppository or liquid or tablet is a "molecular twin" of the progesterone as produced by the ovaries. So in this sense, it may be considered "natural" but it is far from being created by Nature in your own body!

According to various reports, taking progesterone does have its penalties, regardless of whether it eases PMS or not. For example:

- FDA studies with animals show that high doses of progesterone over a period of time may change the body's metabolism and lipid count.
- Synthetic progestogens (note . . . *synthetic!*) were injected into beagle dogs and did cause breast cancer; these progestogens often have adverse effects similar to those of progesterone.
- A suppository often causes a vaginal discharge or leakage. (This may be prevented by using a tampon.)
- A buildup of progesterone may cause the vagina to become dry; this may interfere with sexual relationships. (Doctors suggest insertion of the progesterone suppository after lovemaking.)
- For some women, the added hormone tips the scales so there is a reduced sexual urge; some have a loss of libido. Others say they have stronger urges because of the general feeling of wellbeing.
- The normal menstrual cycle can be affected to induce an early period. Progesterone may also extend menstruation and cause a heavier flow.
- Bleeding disorders during menstruation are among the most reported problems with the use of this substance.
- Progesterone is quickly eliminated by the body. If a woman is on a two-per-day insertion regime (for example) and forgets the program for one day, this immediately provokes a period.
- If the woman continues progesterone beyond the date of her period, the stored up hormonal

supplementation will build up a thick uterine
lining. When treatment is stopped, there could
be reactions of heavy bleeding or hemorrhaging.
Important: Progesterone medication needs to
be taken specifically according to the menstrual
calendar; coordinate it with the anticipated arrival of PMS symptoms.

- Taking progesterone for the first time could induce hot flushes; temporary, but annoying.
- The first-time progesterone user will also have a
  color change in the flow, largely because of a
  reduction in bleeding.
- The vagina reacts to progesterone; there could
  be swelling, yeast infections, vaginal itching.
  Note: these reactions are prompted by the increased levels in progesterone and *not* the type
  of suppository being inserted. You may switch
  to a rectal insert but will still have the symptoms!
- Reports have been cited of such reactions as
  uterine cramps, nausea, irritability, breast tenderness, fatigue and insomnia. These are often
  caused by inappropriate potencies or because
  the medication is not taken at the designated
  times.

Progesterone may need to be taken for a few months
or over many years. Generally, the total dose can be
reduced to a daily minimum and used only the last four
to eight days of the cycle.

Some general statements are offered by Dr. Patricia
Allen on the use of this supplement in her book *Cycles*:

"Dr. Katharina Dalton has reported excellent results
by administering natural progesterone, a substance grown
from yams which is similar to what the body makes on
its own. It is given either by injection or suppository.

"There are no known risks to such treatment so far, except the possible inconvenience of occasional break-through bleeding, and there are reports of 50 to 70 percent of women with initially severe symptoms who claim significant relief within the first month."[49]

Dr. Allen says that "unless your problems are extreme and debilitating, you can probably manage PMS effectively without resorting to expensive hormone therapy.

"In a majority of cases, the right nutritional routine can correct the physiological imbalances—whether too little progesterone, a shortage or surplus of prostaglandins, vitamin or mineral deficiencies or some combination of these—that are causing your discomfort.

"Aerobic and relaxation exercises along with anti-stress techniques will further help keep PMS under control."

VITAMIN B6 TO THE RESCUE

In brief, we see that a hormone imbalance is a major cause of PMS. Estrogen is a cell-proliferating hormone. Progesterone is the antidote for this excess. How can you cause a *natural* production of progesterone which is in short supply and which may be to blame for the symptoms?

Some researchers have suggested vitamin B6 (pyridoxine) as part of a total B-complex supplement program. The importance of this vitamin is explained by Michael G. Brush, M.D., a well-known physician, who tells us, "Inadequate pyridoxine is believed to disrupt the hypothalamus/pituitary connection which can lead to a number of brain-chemical imbalances such as low levels of serotonin, a brain neurotransmitter [low levels of serotonin are a possible cause of depression], and of dopamine [another brain neurotransmitter].

"Too little dopamine can result in an excess of prolactin, a hormone that can adversely affect the ovaries and breasts, and maybe the body's fluid balance as well."[50]

Whatever affects or impairs the proper functioning of the hypothalamus in the brain can result in fluctuating moods, fluid levels, appetite, metabolism. And this same disruption of the hypothalamus can also cause severe premenstrual symptoms.

Both Drs. Allen and Brush agree that the use of pyridoxine together with a prescribed high-potency B-complex tablet could help maintain good hypothalamus/glandular health and bring about reduction or even elimination of symptoms. The vitamin is a *natural* stimulant for progesterone production and that is the name of the game in freedom from PMS!

WILL THE FDA
APPROVE PROGESTERONE?

Actually, in certain forms, and for certain conditions, progesterone is FDA-approved. But the 400-milligram suppositories which Dr. Katharina Dalton recommends for treatment of PMS have not been approved. Why the delay?

Double-blind studies proving the effectiveness of progesterone for treatment of PMS would first have to be conducted for FDA approval. Generally, drug companies recoup the enormous cost of these studies by obtaining long-term patent rights to the drug they are testing. The cost of getting a new drug to market can be as high as $74 million! The patent rights for the process of extracting progesterone ran out twenty years ago. Therefore, no drug company would be able to manufacture the suppositories exclusively. This may explain the reluctance to assume the cost of the double-blind studies.

Consequently, there does not seem to be any possibility of a decision by the FDA, either for or against, and the suppositories will continue to be allowed by individual pharmaceutical preparation, in prescribed dosages. And the risks will still be there! *Caution*: Except for limited use in low dosages (5- or 10-milligram dose injections for irregular periods and uterine bleeding), you use progesterone at your own risk. Since higher dosages are not FDA-approved for PMS, they cannot be shipped across state lines.

NOT A WONDER DRUG

For some women, progesterone may offer the relief they want, but it carries the price of side effects and reactions. For those who have endured PMS for many years, progesterone is not going to completely obliterate past physical, emotional and social problems. It is helpful for some women, less so for others. Only your own reactions and your physician's advice can help you decide whether to use it.

You can stimulate natural progesterone production that will buffer the cramp-causing reactions (among other symptoms) of excess estrogen by using natural methods.

Niels Lauersen, M.D., suggests this basic three-step program:

1. Try applying comfortable heat to painful areas. A heating pad or hot water bottle placed upon your back or on your abdomen can relax the uterus and ease cramps.

2. Try taking vitamins B1 and B6. A suggested combination consists of at least 10 mg of B1 with about 200 mg of B6. This may help regulate your menstrual cycle and lessen the blood buildup in your uterus, thereby lowering the prostaglandin level to help relieve cramping.

3. Exercising regularly will help you shrink fatty tissue,

thereby lessening menstrual flow, lowering prostaglandin levels and boosting progesterone levels. Exercise is also a natural tranquilizer, so it may help relieve tension as it occurs. Try this "comfort pose": Lie on your back and pull your knees close to your chest. Then clasp your knees with your hands and pull them toward your armpits. While in this position, move your feet in a circle.

These three measures will help promote better hormonal balance and freedom from many of the symptoms of PMS . . . naturally.

Chapter 7
HOW TO RELAX AWAY THOSE
STRESSFUL BLUES

PMS was originally dubbed PMT, the last letter standing for "tension." This stressful reaction is one aspect of
the whole syndrome (hence the new name), but it is
one of the most common and most in need of treatment.

The emotional effects of PMS can be devastating;
they include deep depression, tension, anxiety, irritability, fatigue. They can escalate to physical violence. Hormone imbalance can lead to drastic mood swings. It is
therefore useful to try a variety of different methods
that help ease the stressful blues of PMS.

"From the network of PMS sufferers, you hear other
PMS lore almost as grisly," writes Jennifer Allen in
New York magazine. "The woman who tried to drown
her baby, the mother who chased her children around
the house with a .22 because they were getting on her
nerves, suicide attempts, husband beatings, divorces.

"Lives smashed, kaput, because of the invisible beasts
inside them. That's the way women talk about it, too: a
'monster,' a 'Jekyll-and-Hyde' phenomenon."[51]

Dr. Niels H. Lauersen explains why it happens: "When
a woman is under stress, her PMS definitely inten-
sifies. . . . The nervous system and the endocrine, or
hormonal, network in the body make up the neuroendo-

crine system, which is the medical term that defines the complex and sensitive interplays between the brain's nerve signals and the body's fluctuating hormones.

"Nerve-transmitting signals from within the brain affect the release of brain hormones from the hypothalamus and the pituitary, which in turn trigger hormonal action in other parts of the body.

"So although a woman's hormonal imbalance is responsible for the presence of PMS, this imbalance can be traced back to those initial chemical secretions in the brain, signals responding directly to stress. In fact, a high level of stress can inhibit the release of hormones to the point of making the syndrome unbearable."[52]

VITAMINS CAN HELP YOU RELAX . . . NATURALLY

There is a possibility that PMS-related stress could be traced to a deficiency of vitamin A. This was noted by Dr. S. Simkins, an endocrinologist, who used vitamin A as a treatment for overactive thyroid glands. He found, coincidentally, that the use of this vitamin "cured" one woman's premenstrual syndrome. The dosage should be doctor-prescribed for your individual needs, however. And while Dr. Simkins was able to relieve PMS stress with this vitamin, it may or may not be needed for your specific condition.[53]

There has been much research to show that vitamin B6 (pyridoxine) influences premenstrual stress. When you feel tense, depressed, easily agitated or irritated, you may very well have a vitamin B6 deficiency. This is to blame for the decrease in production of dopamine and serotonin, two neurotransmitters or brain chemicals that are needed in correct balance to give you a calm feeling. If you show an estrogen-progesterone imbalance, you are more in need of vitamin B6, which will help stabilize your mood. This nutrient also helps alleviate food cravings and water retention.

Leon Zussman, M.D., diplomate of the American Board of Gynecologists and Obstetricians, and affiliated with the Long Island Jewish–Hillside Medical Center, tells us that "B complex is essential to the health of the liver. And the liver plays a key role in neutralizing the excessive amounts of estrogen produced by the ovaries during the course of the normal menstrual cycle." This means that B6, together with the rest of the members of the B family, could help protect you against the bloating and nervousness that occur premenstrually. [54]

Furthermore, the noted vitamin B6 researcher John M. Ellis, M.D., of Mt. Pleasant, Texas, in his book *The Doctor Who Looked at Hands: Vitamin B6*, lauds this nutrient for being able to relieve that heavy, bloated, puffy feeling so many women experience a week or so prior to menstruation.

A nurse complained to Dr. Ellis that in the midst of her menstrual cycle, she had such swelling of her fingers, she could neither wear rings nor use a typewriter with comfort. Dr. Ellis prescribed 2 50-mg tablets of B6 daily for five days. After two days on this program, the nurse felt improvement. By the third day, she could wear rings, type comfortably and enjoy better sleep. During the next twelve months, she took one 50-mg tablet daily and reportedly was free of PMS pain and swelling. [55]

It is important to consider vitamin E, too, especially because it is believed to have painkilling properties similar to those of aspirin, and it can be obtained in a totally natural form (alpha-tocopherol).

G. E. Desaulniers, M.D., of the famous Shute Institute in London, Ontario, Canada, notes that vitamin E is an excellent weapon against menstrual pain and swelling. It is a mild inhibitor of prostaglandins, as is aspirin, but in most cases has no undesirable side effects. It is also known for being able to improve circulation. Dr. Desaulniers theorizes that menstrual cramps could be caused by a constriction of blood supply when the uterine muscle forcefully contracts. "Where this is the problem," he says, "vitamin E, by promoting better vascular supply, by reducing spasm as it does in other muscle groups throughout the body and by reducing the uterus's need for oxygen, will also reduce the pain resulting from this."[56]

Remember, too, that vitamin E protects against oxidation of fatty substances (vitamin A, essential fatty acids, pituitary, adrenal and sex hormones) and this helps reduce the risk of stress-causing reactions.

CALCIUM HELPS KEEP YOU CALM

This mineral influences the action of muscle fiber by assisting in normal muscle contraction. For instance, if you have ever had muscle cramps or spasms in your calves, you may have noticed that calcium is able to prevent this problem. It is possible that menstrual cramps may be caused by a similar mechanism; after all, the uterus is muscle and menstrual cramps may be caused by excessive contractions of the uterine muscle.

There is also a link between calcium and estrogen. Estrogen helps your body store and use calcium more efficiently. We know this because dwindling estrogen in postmenopausal women leaves them at high risk for the calcium-robbing bone condition called osteoporosis.

Estrogen levels fluctuate cyclically every month. There is a high level that occurs at midcycle when water retention starts. There is a low level prior to your period when cramps and stress are most severe.

Calcium may act as a guardian for estrogen and vice

versa. For many women, the use of calcium carbonate—
preferably with moderate amounts of other vitamins,
and magnesium in a ratio of 1:2 with the calcium—can
ease stress and distress. It may even prevent them!

DR. LAUERSEN'S STRESS SUPPLEMENTATION PROGRAM

Dr. Niels Lauersen says it is important for a woman
"to change the stress-provoking elements in her life in
order to unblock the brain hormones that are preventing her ovaries from producing the needed estrogen
and progesterone."

Dr. Lauersen feels that some vitamin supplementation can help calm a PMS sufferer. He suggests the
following program for relief of PMS stress:

Vitamin E—800-1000 IU a day
Vitamin D—400 IU a day
Calcium—2 to 3 g a day
Vitamin B-complex (with extra B6)—300 to 800
    mg a day
Zinc—50 mg a day
Vitamin C—1000 mg a day

Dr. Lauersen suggests that "by taking extra vitamins
and enrolling in exercise and relaxation programs such
as stretching or yoga classes, a woman may transform the
way her body feels and reverse the course of her PMS."[57]

ELEVEN WAYS TO RELIEVE PMS STRESS

Nutrition should be the foundation of your program
to better health and easing stress before, during and
after menstruation. Remember that your biological
processes are in upheaval. You can be thrown into a
dither over minor problems. You may find it difficult to
get along with others. Anxiety may be driving you up
the wall. With the proper use of nutrition, you can

buffer these reactions. And with some adjustments in your way of living, you can cope with your situation and relieve a great deal of stress.

Try these simple guidelines. Be determined and persistent. The results will be worth your best effort, whether yours is an occasional mild upset, which most of us experience at one time or another, or one that is more lasting and severe. The more you apply these eleven stress-relievers, the more free you will be from PMS.

1. *Talk It Out.* When something worries you, don't bottle it up. Confide your worry to some levelheaded person you can trust—your husband, father or mother, a good friend, your clergyman, your family doctor, a teacher, school counselor or dean. Talking things out helps to relieve your strain, helps you to see your worry in a clearer light, and often helps you to see what you can do about it.

2. *Escape for a While.* Sometimes when things go wrong, it helps to escape from the painful problem *for a while*, to lose yourself in a movie, book or game, or a brief trip for a change of scene. Making yourself "stand there and suffer" is a form of self-punishment, not a way to solve a problem. It is perfectly realistic and healthy to want to escape punishment long enough to recover breath and balance. But be prepared to come back and deal with your difficulty when you are more composed, and when you and others involved are better prepared to deal with it.

3. *Work off Your Anger.* If you feel yourself using anger as a general mode of behavior, remember that while anger may give you a temporary sense of righteousness, or even of power, it will generally leave you feeling foolish and sorry in the end. If you feel like lashing out at someone who has provoked you, try

holding off that impulse for a while. Let it wait until tomorrow. Meanwhile, do something constructive with your pent-up energy. Pitch into some physical activity like gardening, cleaning out the garage, carpentry or a do-it-yourself project. Or work it out in tennis or a brisk walk. Working the anger out of your system and cooling it off for a day or two will leave you much better prepared to handle your problem.

4. *Give in Occasionally*. If you find yourself getting into frequent quarrels with people, and feeling obstinate and defiant, remember that that's the way frustrated children behave. Stand your ground on what you know is right, but do so calmly and make allowance for the fact that you *could* turn out to be wrong. And even if you're dead right, it's easier on your system to give in once in awhile. If you yield, you'll usually find that others will, too. And if you can work it out, the result will be relief from tension, the achievement of a practical solution, together with a great feeling of satisfaction and maturity.

5. *Do Something for Others*. If you feel yourself worrying about yourself all the time, try doing something for somebody else. You'll find this will take the steam out of your own worries and—even better—give you the satisfaction of having done well.

6. *Take One Thing at a Time*. For women suffering from PMS, an ordinary work load can sometimes seem unbearable. The load looks so great that it becomes painful to tackle any part of it—even the things that most need to be done. When that happens, remember that it's a temporary condition and that you can work your way out of it. The surest way to do this is to take a few of the most urgent tasks and pitch into them, one at a time, setting aside all the rest for the time being. Once you dispose of these you'll see that the remainder

is not so overwhelming after all. You'll be in the swing of things, and the rest of the tasks will go much more easily. If you feel you can't set *any*thing aside in this sensible way, reflect: are you sure you aren't overestimating the importance of the things you do—that is, your own importance?

7. *Shun the "Superwoman" Urge.* Some PMS sufferers expect too much from themselves, and get into a constant state of anxiety because they think they are not achieving as much as they should. They try for perfection in everything. Admirable as this attempt is, it is an open invitation to failure. No one can be perfect in everything. Decide which things you do well, and put your major effort into these. They are apt to be the things you like to do and, hence, those that give you the most satisfaction. Then, perhaps, come the things you can't do so well. Give them the best of your effort and ability, but don't take yourself to task if you can't achieve the impossible.

8. *Go Easy with Your Criticism.* Some people expect too much of others and then feel frustrated, let down, disappointed, even "trapped" when another person does not measure up. The "other person" may be a husband or a child whom we are trying to fit into a preconceived pattern—perhaps even trying to make over to suit ourselves. Remember, each person has his own virtues, his own shortcomings, his own values, his own right to develop as an individual. If you feel let down by the shortcomings (real or imagined) of others, you are really let down about yourself. Instead of being critical of the other person's behavior, search out his good points and help him to develop them. This will give both of you satisfaction and help you to gain a better perspective on yourself as well.

9. *Give the Other Fellow a Break.* When you are

under PMS tension, you often feel you have to "get there first"—to edge out the other person, even if the goal is as trivial as getting ahead on the highway. If enough feel that way—and many do—then everything becomes a race in which somebody is bound to get injured—physically, as on the highway, or emotionally and mentally, in the effort to live a full life. It need not be this way. Competition is contagious, but so is cooperation. When you give the other person a break, you very often make things easier for yourself; if he no longer feels you are a threat, then he stops being a threat to you.

10. *Make Yourself "Available."* Many women during PMS have the feeling of being "left out," slighted, neglected, rejected. Often, you just imagine that other people feel this way about you, when in reality they are eager for you to make the first move. Most likely, you (not the others) are deprecating yourself. Instead of shrinking away and withdrawing, it is much healthier, as well as more practical, to continue to "make yourself available"—to make some of the overtures instead of always waiting to be asked. Of course, the opposite of withdrawal—pushing yourself forward on every occasion—is equally futile. This is often misinterpreted and may lead to real rejection. There is a middle ground. Try it.

11. *Schedule Your Recreation.* Many people drive themselves so hard that they allow themselves too little time for recreation—an essential for good physical and mental health during PMS. You may find it hard to make yourself take time out. If so, a set routine and schedule will help—a program of definite hours when you will engage in some recreation. And in general it is desirable for you to have a hobby that absorbs you in off hours, one into which you can throw yourself com-

pletely and with pleasure, forgetting all about your responsibilities.

According to the National Mental Health Association, which helped prepare this eleven-step stress-easing program, it is also soothing to have faith in yourself and in others. But if you find that PMS still gives you the willies, you should seek help from a specialist who is able to help you cope with the situation.[58]

QUICK WAYS TO
REDUCE STRESS FURTHER

Once you know you have PMS, you can quickly and easily reduce the risk of stress by making your life more simplified during the cycle.

For example, postpone housecleaning until you are free of the symptoms. An exception may be an urge to do sudden cleaning right then and there and this could be good therapy.

Ask your youngsters and/or husband to help in the everyday chores such as shopping, washing dishes, even cooking.

If you have some meetings scheduled, try to postpone them until you are able to cope with the responsibilities involved. If not, tackle just one or two of the most important ones.

Having a dinner party? Does it conflict with your period? Keep a careful calendar. Mark those days during which your symptoms are worst and avoid stressful social activities during that time.

Prepare a list of tasks; do only the most necessary ones. Postpone whatever can be delayed. Get into the habit of saying, "Sorry, not this week" or "A week later." No need to tell everyone (except those who understand) that you have PMS. It is, after all, a personal situation.

Be realistic. Things can upset you easily; prepare for this. Be honest and tell yourself that you may overreact because of your glandular upheaval. Give yourself a pep talk—out loud, if need be. Bolster your ego. Convince yourself that "This too shall pass." A little self-encouragement and a pat on the back can work wonders. You will be able to meet daily challenges before, during and after your period with this self-assurance.

You cannot build a life completely free of stress, with or without PMS. So it is important for you to develop ways of dealing with stress. Be grateful for one biological fact. PMS is predictable. You know when it will happen. You can prepare for it. You can deal with it successfully.

Chapter 8
FITNESS FOR PMS CONTROL

FEEL LIKE CLIMBING THE WALLS? You're in the throes of
PMS. Don't just sit there—get moving! Fitness can
help tame those hormonal reactions. Physical activity
releases the tension created by stress. As oxygen enters
your lungs, your heart pumps, your blood circulates
and your hormones become "unchained" and flow more
freely. You feel good all over.

Furthermore, exercise not only eases the pain of
PMS while you are in its grip, but if performed daily, it
can help protect against cramps and other menstrual
complaints before they begin.

According to the President's Council on Fitness, seven
or eight out of every ten women who have PMS are also
negligent when it comes to exercise. According to the
Council, exercise works in many ways to relieve reactions commonly associated with PMS. Exercise will relieve constipation by increasing intestinal contractions.
It helps protect against that waterlogged feeling by
helping you get rid of fluids through a good sweat. It
also prompts healthy deep breathing, important in bring-
ing more oxygen to your blood. (This helps relax your
uterus so you have fewer painful contractions.) Exercise
eases stress-tension-depression by causing an increase

of endorphins and other hormones to help you cheer up.

Whatever exercises your major muscle groups, gets you breathing and creates an oxygenation of your system will protect against cramps and other symptoms of PMS. Consider jogging, swimming, cycling, fast-paced walking, Dancercise. Consider stretching exercises for your hips and lower back. Sit-ups, too, are helpful. Eight weeks of the bent-knee variety done on a daily basis were found to make life much easier during PMS for thirty-six college women tested by a team of physicians.[59] Easy, enjoyable, effective!

AEROBICS ARE TOPS
FOR PMS RELIEF

Any sustained, vigorous exercise that gets and keeps your pulse rate up is beneficial; aerobics are always considered best. This is a form of oxygenation that conditions your cardiovascular system but also enables your body to metabolize carbohydrates more thoroughly.

Aerobic exercise will also help release beta-endorphins, those natural morphine-like substances in your body that can calm your moods. With regular exercise, you will have less fluid and sodium retention. You will also stimulate a sleepy digestive system and pep up your stomach muscles. Exercise will help body tensions evaporate, relieve muscular aches and help you sleep better. Aerobics with stretching will also keep your muscles more flexible; this reduces susceptibility to cramping pain.

Aim to have your pulse rate rise to 80 percent of your aerobic training level. This is your "target zone." Calculate by subtracting your age from 220 (your maximum pulse-heart rate). Thus, a thirty-year-old woman should try to get her heart rate to 80 percent of 190 or about

152 beats per minute during the time she is working out.

To see if you are within your target zone, take your pulse immediately after you stop exercising. (You'll find your pulse on the inside of your wrist just below the base of your thumb.) Count your pulse for 30 seconds and then multiply by two. Once you're exercising within your target zone, check your pulse at least once each week during the first three months and periodically thereafter.

BEFORE YOU BEGIN

If you have been a weekend athlete or sedentary for a long time, you need first to check with your physician to establish a desirable starting level. Then you can make appropriate schedules for fitness.

If you've been inactive for a while, you may want to start with brisk walking or swimming, rather than jogging or jumping rope. Beginning with less strenuous activities will allow you to become more fit without straining your body. Once you have gotten into better shape, you can progress to more vigorous activity.

Select a time slot and stick to it. Then plan to exercise from thirty to forty minutes at a time. That's all there is to it. You should notice important benefits in very short order.

A warm-up period is crucial to the success and safety of any exercise program. A good warm-up is essential to elevate your heart rate and respiration, increase your circulation, promote blood vessel dilation and raise body temperature. Simple stretching relieves stress and tension in your muscles, making them more pliable so they can do more with less risk of hurt.

Stretching Is a Good Warm-Up. Just 10 minutes of stretching before your regular exercise will warm up your body. Stretching is fun and it prepares you for the exercise to follow. Try some of these stretches:

Stretch Neck, Upper Spine. Stand straight. Relax your shoulders. Gently roll head to the right, touching ear close to shoulder, then back as far as is comfortably possible (letting your mouth hang open) to your left shoulder. Repeat several times, back and forth.

Shoulders, Upper Back, Chest, Neck. Use a slow, smooth motion. Roll your shoulders all the way forward; now all the way up, back, then down. Repeat in reverse direction.

Stretch Lower Back, Hips. Lie on your back, legs straight, feet relaxed. Raise one knee and hold with fingers. Gently press knee toward your chest. Keep the other leg flat on floor. Hold; release slowly. Repeat with other knee.

Stretch Back of Legs, Lower Back. Sit on floor; extend legs straight to front. Keep back straight and feet flexed. Slowly bend and reach over legs. Take hold of your ankles. Gently bring forehead toward legs as far as it is comfortable to do so. Hold for the count of five. Slowly curl up from lower back. Repeat three times.

Stretch Entire Body. Lie flat on your back. Keep legs straight, stomach down. Lower your back and press to the floor. Extend arms behind your head. Point your toes. Give yourself a long, total body stretch as far as you can. *Tip*: Pretend you are on a "rack" and being pulled from both directions. Hold and slowly release. Repeat several times.

REMEMBER: YOU MUST KEEP BREATHING NORMALLY DURING ALL OF THESE AND OTHER EXERCISES.

After your exercise session, let your body cool down slowly. You need to give your heart, lungs and muscles a chance to adjust after exercise.

Do some more mild stretching and deep breathing; try walking while you swing your arms. All help you cool down. You can also cool down by changing to a less vigorous exercise, such as going from jumping rope to walking, swimming more slowly or changing to a more leisurely stroke. This allows your body to relax gradually.

Caution: Abrupt stopping can cause dizziness. If you have been running, walking briskly or jumping rope, repeat your stretching and limbering exercises to loosen up your muscles.

STRESS-EASING EXERCISES

Wall Push-Aways

- Stand facing a wall, an arm's length away.
- Inhale as you bend arms and lower your body to the wall. Allow heels to lift off floor.
- Exhale as you push back to standing position.
- Repeat 15 to 30 times.

Abdominals

- Sit with knees bent, hands resting on knees and chin tucked in to chest.
- Exhale as you s-l-o-w-l-y lower down: first back, then shoulders, then head to touch floor.
- Knees remain bent throughout.
- Use arms to assist return to sitting position.
- Repeat five times.

Curl-Up

- Lie on back, knees bent, feet flat on floor, arms relaxed at sides.
- Press small of back flat to the floor.
- Lift head and shoulders off floor and look toward knees while exhaling.
- Relax and repeat up to five times.

Single-Knee Tuck

- Lie on back, one leg straight and one leg bent.
- Keeping bent leg still, grasp hands behind the other knee and pull it toward your chest while exhaling. Hold.
- Alternate legs and repeat.
- Your lower back and head remain on the floor throughout.
- Repeat up to 15 times.

Side Leg Raises (For thighs, hips and waist)

- Lie on one side with head resting comfortably on extended arm, the other arm and hand resting on floor in front of your waist (to maintain balance).
- Bottom leg should be bent at your knee to protect your back.
- Exhale as you slowly raise top leg; inhale as you slowly lower it.
- Top leg should remain straight and toes should point forward throughout.
- Repeat on other side.

Soothing Exercise

- Lie on your back, knees bent and legs resting on a couch or chair.
- Rest your head on a folded towel, back flat to floor and hands resting comfortably on your abdomen.
- Breathe quietly with no effort to inhale deeply until you feel completely relaxed.
- As you take a slightly deeper breath, let your abdomen rise; then s-l-o-w-l-y exhale through pursed lips, letting your abdomen relax downward.
- Repeat as desired.

Side Bends

- Stand with feet wide apart.
- S-l-o-w-l-y reach one arm down the outside of your leg while exhaling. Hold.
- Repeat to the other side.
- May also be done sitting: hold side edge of chair with one hand and reach down to the other side.

Caution: If you are experiencing back pain, omit this exercise and check with your physician.

Simple Squats

- Stand with your feet shoulder-width apart; arms extended out to each side.
- Crouch or squat with your back straight and reach down with both arms between your legs.
- Return to start by extending legs.
- Repeat five times.

It is essential for you to stretch your spine, with its delicate nerve endings, to strengthen your back and abdomen, and to send nutrient-carrying blood circulating throughout your reproductive organs. In so doing, you will be able to ease the distress of PMS. The preceding exercises (remember the warm-up and cooldown) are aimed at reducing the incidence of mental and physical stress. Follow them regularly and you should find immeasurable relief from PMS.

HOW TO BECOME MORE ACTIVE THROUGHOUT THE DAY

Take advantage of any opportunity to get up and move around. Here are some examples:

- Use the stairs—up and down—instead of the elevator. Start with one flight of stairs and gradually build up to more.

- Park a few blocks from the office or store and walk the rest of the way. Or if you use public transportation, get off a stop or two before and walk the remaining few blocks.
- Take an exercise break—get up and stretch frequently. Walk around. Give your muscles and mind a chance to relax.
- Instead of eating that extra snack, take a brisk stroll around the neighborhood.
- Stand, instead of sitting, whenever you can.
- Clean your house or apartment often. This can be excellent exercise.
- Instead of going to dinner or a movie some evening, go dancing. It's a great way to oxygenate and activate your entire body.

WALK YOUR WAY TO FITNESS

Walking is an easy and effective aerobic exercise. It activates your muscles, improves circulation in your legs, hips and pelvic area (where congestion is part of PMS), stimulates elimination and melts away tension.

All you need do is wear comfortable shoes (running shoes are best) and loose clothing. Walk with your whole body. Keep your back straight and tall, your tummy tucked in, your shoulders relaxed. Swing your legs from your hips in long strides. Keep your arms loose and let them swing naturally.

You need to have a brisk walk, not a leisurely one that is too "sedentary" and does not oxygenate your system. Plan to walk briskly at a rate of one mile every 15 minutes (about 175 feet every 30 seconds). Aim for half a mile (10 city blocks). Alternate one block of brisk walking with one block at a slower pace. Your ultimate goal is to walk one hour (4 miles) a day, 5 days a week.

ARE YOU A JOGGER?

To begin, you first have to check with your doctor, especially if you are overweight or over thirty. If you have approval, then plan to jog.

Choose a good pair of running shoes that have arch support, firm support at the heel, about one inch of good padding under the heel and a high toe box. Clothes should be comfortable, porous and either warm for cold weather or cool for warm weather.

Running is done with your body upright; keep hips in line with your shoulders. Arms need to be bent with forearms parallel to the ground. Keep hands at waist level, comfortably clenched.

Lift legs from your thighs. Hit your heel on the ground and roll to your forefoot. NEVER run on the balls of your feet because you will strain your calf muscles.

Begin slowly. You could start with brisk walking, then alternate with jogging. Do each for 30 to 60 seconds at a time. Aim for 5 minutes at the start. Gradually progress to straight jogging. Increase your distance, day to day, week to week. *Goal*: Just 20 minutes of jogging, 5 days a week.

Remember, you don't have to run fast. You're not in a race. It's the distance that matters.

Turn jogging into fun. Do it with a friend. Join a club. Meet fellow runners along the way. Plan a run as part of an afternoon outing. Explore new locations.

TRY JUMPING ROPE

It's like having a traveling gym—easy to pack and use anywhere. Don't jump with both feet at once. That could shock your body. Instead, find a soft surface (grass or carpet) and alternate from foot to foot as you jump. It's not too easy to jump rope for 12 minutes, so you need to work into this exercise by conditioning with other activities first.

Tip: Keep your chin up. Jump like a boxer in training. Use tennis shoes. When you stand on the middle of the rope, each handle should come up to your armpit. This is the way to select a good rope.

WHEELS AWAY

Bicycling is a great aerobic exercise; it doesn't jar your body because your weight is not supported by your feet. You should plan to bicycle as much as you can; throughout the day, time permitting, wherever possible. You could stow your bike in the car, drive out to the country or nearest bicycle trail or even to a school campus. It makes bicycling so much more interesting.

The same guidelines for fitness apply to a cycling program: use a warm-up–cool-down pattern. Aim for 20 minutes, three non-consecutive days or more.

AEROBIC DANCING

You don't need to go outside. Instead, turn on some brisk music at home, do your chores and dance around from room to room. Dig up some records with peppy songs for at least 12 minutes. Make up a routine of steps for yourself. Just remember to check your pulse rate and adjust your pace accordingly.

Tip: Use tennis shoes for aerobic dancing at home, not running shoes, because they are not made for sideways motion and can cause problems if used for dancing.

BENCH STEPPING

Very simply, this calls for stepping up and down repeatedly on a bench or on one step of a staircase. Try it to snappy music. It helps establish a rhythm and turns this exercise into an upbeat experience.

To bench step, just step up with your right foot, bring your left foot up on to the bench, step down with your right foot and then bring your left foot down. Alternate your leading foot with each set. Your heart rate is determined by the height of the bench or chair which you are using. If your bench stepping heart rate is too high, find a lower bench!

SWIMMING

This is a great exercise for stretching your muscles, reducing the distress of PMS-caused cramping. It gives you a marvelous feeling when you glide through the water. But like all aerobic exercises, it has to be regular to be effective.

Swim in the longest available pool so you don't need to do much turning. Alternate swimming with other aerobics for variety. Plan to swim as often as possible. (Wear a brightly colored bathing suit to make you feel even better!)

HOW LONG SHOULD YOU EXERCISE?

Each session should last from about 25 to 40 minutes and include:

> 5 minutes—warm up
> 15-30 minutes—exercising in your target zone
> 5 minutes—cool down

That's all there is to it. Surely, this modest amount of time spent on alternate days is a small price to pay for helping to condition your body so that you have greater resistance to the effects of hormonal imbalance.

MORE HELPFUL TIPS

- If you've eaten a meal, avoid exercise for at least 2 hours. If you exercise vigorously first, wait about 20 minutes before eating.

- Use proper equipment, such as good running shoes with adequate cushioning in the soles.
- Jogging on hard or uneven surfaces such as cement or rough ground is more likely to cause injuries. Soft, even surfaces such as a level grass field, a dirt path, or a track are better for your feet, joints and body.
- If you run or jog, land on your heels rather than the balls of your feet. This will minimize the strain on your feet and lower legs.
- Joggers or walkers should also watch for cars and wear light-colored clothes or a reflecting band at night so that drivers can see them. Face oncoming traffic and do not assume that drivers will notice you on the roadway.
- If you bicycle, you can help prevent injuries by wearing a helmet and using a light and reflectors on the wheels at night. Also, ride in the direction of traffic. Try to avoid busy streets.

With a regular fitness program, you can help tame your glandular reactions and ease the distress of PMS—perhaps even eradicate it.

Chapter 9
MENSTRUAL CRAMPS: NEW SOURCES OF RELIEF

PROSTAGLANDINS are hormone-like substances found in every cell in your body. They are a remarkable family of chemical messengers that participate in many of your life processes. It is believed that one group of prostaglandins is responsible for the symptoms associated with PMS.

Prostaglandins are so named because they were first isolated from prostate gland secretions, but they are found everywhere, including the uterus, where they affect contraction and relaxation. They exert powerful effects in quantities as small as one *billionth* of a gram.

Prostaglandins are vital. They cause contractions of the smooth involuntary muscles of the body, such as the blood vessels, intestines, heart and uterus. They are often used to stimulate labor contractions.

In women, prostaglandins are manufactured by the uterus just prior to and during the onset of menstruation. (This accounts for the cramping and aches felt premenstrually and during the first day or so of the period.) They are needed because the unused endometrial lining must be shed each cycle so that a fresh lining can be created for the next egg. Prostaglandins produce the contractions that are necessary to expel the unused uterine lining.

Prostaglandins are being tested as healers for various ailments such as leg ulcers, Raynaud's disease (gangrene) and a form of angina that occurs when the person is at rest. These substances (considered to be unsaturated fatty acids) have been found to help in conditions such as arthritis, cardiovascular disorders, hypertension or high blood pressure, excessive cholesterol, breast lumps and eczema.

It is an *excess* of prostaglandins that causes intense menstrual pain. Furthermore, high levels of prostaglandins may cause nausea, irritability and water retention, among other PMS symptoms. Speaking simply, too many prostaglandins cause the uterus to contract too often and too hard. This leads to painful spasms and uterine cramps. This is worsened when the severely contracted uterine muscle compresses its own blood vessels and cuts off its blood supply, intensifying the pain. PMS specialist Penny Wise Budoff, M.D., clinical associate professor of family medicine at the State University of New York at Stony Brook, likens this situation to the cutting off of blood from the heart. "It is similar to a situation when the heart goes into spasms during a heart attack." She describes how excruciating the pain (angina) can be. Dr. Budoff also suggests that there would be a better understanding of menstrual pain if it were renamed "uterine angina."[60]

THE ROUTE OF THE PROSTAGLANDINS

Cramp-causing prostaglandins are usually controlled by the hormone progesterone. But prior to menstruation, there is a drop in progesterone and a corresponding rise in prostaglandins. The mouth of the womb (cervix), from which the blood usually flows, now constricts.

Prostaglandins in the menstrual blood locked within the womb are absorbed by the uterine muscles and a vicious cycle begins. The prostaglandins are released, reabsorbed, released again in a circular manner. The pain is ready to begin.[61]

As the prostaglandins go their route, the uterus tightens and cramps more severely. The pain will continue until the menstrual blood is discharged from the vagina, carrying along the prostaglandins. But even as the prostaglandins are discharged, the uterus contracts and cramps. This causes what is often considered a "charley horse" of the womb. At times, these uterine contractions can be sharper than labor pains.

If the blood cannot escape through the vagina, there is a backup, starting in the fallopian tubes, then into the abdominal cavity. This worsens the already unbearable cramps and may predispose a woman to endometriosis, a disease in which the tissue that constitutes the uterine lining (endometrium) spreads to other organs.

It is important for you *not* to wait too long before seeing a physician if you have these severe menstrual pains. While you may cope with the pain, you may have a serious ailment such as an infection or pelvic disease in need of medical treatment.

Unlike systemic hormones, prostaglandins are local messengers; they influence only the part of the body where they are made. For example, one group regulates blood clotting, another contracts blood vessels and smooth muscles, another group influences intestinal motions, a different one is involved in heartbeat and another set controls breathing.

But there is another set that is to blame for the pain, swelling and inflammation of arthritis. There is still another that constricts the walls of blood vessels close to the heart to set off the agonizing chest pains of angina. And the most familiar is the prostaglandin group released by the endometrium that forces the smooth-muscle tissue to contract, resulting in menstrual spasms.

According to researchers W. Y. Chan and M. Yusoff Dawood of New York's Cornell University Medical College, women troubled with painful periods have two or three times the level of prostaglandins in their menstrual fluid of those who are free of symptoms. The doctors note that these high concentrations are to blame for more frequent, powerful and longer-lasting contractions, along with higher pressures within the uterus; these are felt as spasmodic, labor-like pain. They explain that this discomfort radiates to the back, along the thighs and legs as well, justifying the name of "syndrome." Furthermore, the excessive overload of prostaglandins reacts upon local nerve endings, making them more sensitive to pain.[62]

WHY PROSTAGLANDINS ARE IMPORTANT

Researchers have found that while some prostaglandins are to blame for the painful contractions, others in the body are essential to bodily processes. And this presents a problem for the prostaglandin-inhibitors: along with blocking the "bad" ones, they block the "good" ones. This probably accounts for the side effects experienced. This finding has led a number of scientists to suggest that it would be healthier to inhibit only the "bad" prostaglandins. You do need the "good" ones.

EIGHT IMPORTANT FUNCTIONS OF PROSTAGLANDINS

The well-known British gynecologist Caroline Shreeve, M.D., explains that prostaglandin E1 is necessary for a number of functions, such as:

1. To prevent thrombosis and lower blood pressure.
2. To open up blood vessels and relieve angina.
3. To slow down the speed with which cholesterol is made.
4. To enable insulin to work more efficiently.
5. To prevent inflammation and control arthritis.
6. To perpetrate different actions on the brain; in humans, it produces a sense of wellbeing.
7. Under laboratory conditions, to stop cancer cells from growing.
8. To relieve the physical and mental symptoms of the premenstrual syndrome.[63]

The intricacies of this process were first discovered by a brilliant young British-born doctor and pioneer in PG (prostaglandin) research, David Horrobin. He is a former professor of medicine at the University of Montreal, and later became completely involved in research in the field of prostaglandins and the use of evening primrose oil as a natural healer.

There are two types of prostaglandins. One is "good," the second is hurtful. "Not all PGs are alike," says Dr. Horrobin, "and it is vital for you to stimulate your body so that it releases an abundance of the *good* variety. It may be a hairline difference but it makes a world of difference in terms of mental and physical health."[64]

According to Dr. Horrobin, "The level of PGE1 is of crucial importance to the body. A fall in the level of PGE1 will lead to a potentially catastrophic series of untoward consequences, including increased vascular reactivity, enhanced blood clotting, elevated cholesterol production, diabetic-like changes in insulin release, enhanced risk of auto-immune disease, enhanced risk of inflammatory disorders and susceptibility to depression."[65]

Adequate levels of PGE1 are also necessary for normal function of the T-cells (T suppressor lymphocytes) of the immune system (they reject foreign invaders capable of causing infection). In addition, PGE1 influences the release of substances from nerve cells that transmit nerve impulses and it regulates the movement of soothing calcium in the cells.

The problem with taking a chemotherapeutic anti-prostaglandin medicine is, as we have said, that you are blocking the *good* PGs along with the *bad* ones. Therefore, you may be blocking out pain, but you are also inhibiting essential bodily processes. Furthermore, a shortage of PGE1 coupled with an excess of prolactin may cause cystic mastitis (also known as benign breast disease or fibrocystic disease of the breast, which affects two out of every ten premenopausal women). This condition may also be brought on by using anti-prostaglandin medicines. That is, when you induce a shortage of protective PGE1, your body becomes vulnerable to the effects of prolactin.

Dr. Horrobin discovered that the body's ability to manufacture PGE1 (the "good" PG) can be triggered by only two foods in Nature: mother's milk, and the oil from a common plant, evening primrose.

EVENING PRIMROSE OIL TO THE RESCUE

A member of the dicotyledonous plant family (*Oenothera biennis*), evening primrose is a beautiful, tall wild plant. In late summer, it produces a long spike of primrose-like yellow flowers that open in the evening; hence its name. Other varieties have different colors. Generally, the plants range from two to five feet in height. They bloom in the evening, at which time they are pollinated by night-flying insects. The delicate flowers survive just one night, then wither to a pinkish tinge. The plants are biennials and require two years to bloom, then die in the fall.

The American Indians made medicines from all parts of this plant for the healing of skin diseases, wounds and choking symptoms (today known as asthma). Their knowledge was shared with the Pilgrims, who used the plant as a natural medicine. According to researcher M. Moore of the University of New Mexico, "Chief Two-Trees of the Cherokee nation has found evening primrose to lessen spasms, to be used as a sedative, pain killer, diuretic and a mild astringent. The root is used for making a cough syrup that is especially effective against whooping cough, asthmatic cough and TB cough. The sedative effect varies with the species and with the person. This effect is due to the potassium nitrate found in all parts of the plant."[66]

As early as 1614, American colonists introduced it in England, where it became known as the King's Cure-All. Particularly valued were the very tiny dark brown seeds which were said to contain the ingredients that produce the healing effects. These seeds contain a unique nutrient, gamma-linolenic acid or GLA (which is abundant in only one other food, human milk), which creates your body's supply of PGE1, the "good" prostaglandin that is needed for protection against illness.

For relief of PMS, your goal is to prompt the manufacture of PGE1, but not of excess PGE2, the hurtful PG. You need essential fatty acids, particularly linoleic acid, which is usually found in vegetable oils such as sunflower and safflower, especially the latter. The oil is converted first to gammalinolenic acid (GLA) and then to dihomogammalinolenic acid (DGLA) and finally to PGE1.

But the ability to form GLA can be impeded by a lack of essential fatty acids, deficiencies of zinc, vitamin

B6 and magnesium, as well as by virus infections, alcohol, and the aging process. Therefore, the goal is to find a natural source of GLA, the substance that will eventually become healing PGE1. One such source is the seed oil of the evening primrose.

Vegetable oils are not a good alternative because while they do contain essential fatty acids and the needed linoleic acid, oils go through so many complex refining processes that their effectiveness is diminished. "During these processes," says Dr. Horrobin, "much of the linoleic acid becomes converted into trans acids that cannot be properly used by the body.

"Unless linoleic acid can be converted into GLA, it cannot be of much help to your body. Therefore, you are given fewer GLAs, if any, and your production of PGE1 falls down. This creates a deficiency and your body becomes vulnerable to ailments. This is why the oil from evening primrose is so valuable. It provides the GLA *directly*, [thus] bypassing the block in body chemistry."[67]

PGE1 is vulnerable to an onslaught of other influences known as blockers. These include "trans fat," saturated (animal) fats, alcohol, virus infections and cancer. Trans fats are a byproduct of partially or fully hydrogenated fats. They block the formation of the PGE1 group and this makes the body all the more vulnerable to PMS, among other illnesses. A rule of thumb here would be to avoid processed foods containing these objectionable trans fats. These include margarine, breadings, cakes, candies, cookies, nondairy creamers, pastries, pies, puddings, shortenings, doughnuts, fried crusts and frostings, to name just a few.

Niels H. Lauersen, M.D., has this to say about evening primrose oil:

"A woman who takes an evening primrose capsule

provides her body with linoleic acid for the increase of the PGE1 [good] prostaglandin. [Linoleic acid is also naturally contained in vegetable oils such as cold-pressed safflower oil.] PGE1 lowers blood pressure, prevents blood clots and may lower cholesterol levels and strengthen the immune system. It has been experimentally used as a treatment for alcoholism, eczema, schizophrenia, and as a hangover remedy. Not all of the claims for PGE1 have been proved but the research continues."[68]

Why is evening primrose oil helpful? Dr. David Horrobin believes the oil may influence symptoms that originate from the activity of the hormone prolactin. This hormone, synthesized and stored in the pituitary gland, stimulates production of progesterone by the ovaries; an excessive secretion of prolactin means more progesterone and more pain. Dr. Horrobin suggests that symptoms may depend on how the linoleic acid levels react with prolactin activity. It is believed that "the steady production of PGE1, which can be maintained with the linoleic acid of the evening primrose oil, may suppress PMS symptoms stemming from prolactin."[69]

A treatment with evening primrose oil was administered by Dr. M. G. Brush of the Premenstrual Syndrome Clinic in London's St. Thomas's Hospital Medical School. Dr. Brush gave the oil to sixty-five PMS sufferers; other treatments had not helped. At the end of the study, 61 percent of the women had total relief, while 23 percent had partial relief.[70] There were no side effects reported; this is to be expected because evening primrose oil is a natural product. Furthermore, since evening primrose oil stimulates release of PGE1 but not PGE2, it does *not* block total PGE production, hence does not change basic biological processes.

Dr. Horrobin has found that this oil is by far the richest natural source of biologically active essential fatty acids needed to initiate the chain reaction to culminate in PGE1. "It contains about 72 percent of cis-linoleic acid (the active component form) and about 9 percent of GLA. Four out of five women with PMS reported an amazing improvement with evening primrose oil. Also, some women with painful, lumpy breasts also reported relief of pain and a lessening of the discomfort."[71]

Michael Schachter, M.D., a nutritionally oriented physician from Nyack, New York, also uses evening primrose oil as part of natural treatment for PMS patients. "I've been using it on patients for a year or two. It seems to help very much in cases of premenstrual syndrome.

"I also prescribe the cofactors of evening primrose oil—that is, magnesium, zinc, vitamin B6 and niacin. In addition, patients are asked to reduce their consumption of saturated fat just before their periods and also to reduce sugar.

"Patients who do this, along with taking 3 to 4 grams of evening primrose oil a day, usually get significant relief. In fact, I have seen an 80 to 90 percent improvement among patients who suffer from premenstrual syndrome when they follow this program."[72]

NOT ALL PRODUCTS ARE ALIKE

According to Edward Perkins, Ph.D., who tested any number of products, "There's a good chance that someone buying evening primrose oil will not be getting the product she paid for. Of all the samples I've analyzed, almost 30 percent have been found lacking any GLA. Instead, they contain soybean oil, maybe mixed with another oil. Moreover, evening primrose oil should contain six to eight percent GLA, but I've seen some samples with only one or two percent, which makes you suspicious."[73]

According to Ann Nazzaro, Ph.D., a psychobiologist in practice in Northampton, Massachusetts, with PMS specialist Donald Lombard, M.D., the product should be made from the seeds, *not* from cheaper leaves, which do not contain enough GLA to do any good. "A lot of women on primrose oil suddenly complain that their symptoms have returned and we find that they've switched to a cheaper brand." Dr. Nazzaro's advice is to use a well-known brand which contains standardized amounts of oil from commercially cultivated hybrid plants rich in GLA. A typical capsule should have 500 milligram strength. The usual dose for symptoms is 6 to 8 500-milligram capsules daily. After several months, you should be able to get along on a much lower maintenance dose. "There's nothing magical about evening primrose oil," says Dr. Nazzaro. "It simply corrects a chemical imbalance."[74]

Read labels. Make certain the product contains gamma-linolenic acid, the ingredient which makes it effective.

Prostaglandins are very short-lived body chemicals. They are continuously made by the body just when and where they are needed. They are destroyed as soon as they have served their immediate purpose. You cannot afford to let your body become deficient in the important PGE1 variety. By using evening primrose oil, you can help relieve the symptoms of premenstrual syndrome.

OVER-THE-COUNTER RELIEF FOR CRAMPS

Some over-the-counter products have long been used for relief of menstrual cramps. Let's examine each of these in terms of their usefulness and possible side effects.

Aspirin (acetylsalicylic acid). This popular drug is used to relieve pain and also reduce inflammation and fever. It works as an anti-prostaglandin agent and anticoagulant, which may protect against pain associated with clots passing through the cervical opening during menstruation. Some doctors recommend taking aspirin a few days before the period to inhibit prostaglandin production.

Caution: Aspirin may irritate the lining of the stomach, causing nausea, pain and bleeding. High doses cause dizziness, disturbed hearing, mental confusion and hyperventilation. Ulcerous patients should not use it since it induces stomach bleeding. Ringing in the ears may be another side effect. Buffered aspirin has a small amount of antacid added. This enables it to be absorbed faster and reduces the adverse affects of plain aspirin. Diuretics containing ammonium chloride and large doses of vitamin C may conflict with aspirin and slow its elimination from your body, which may give you prolonged gastric irritation.

Acetaminophen. An aspirin substitute favored by those who cannot take aspirin. This drug works as an anticoagulant but does not cause stomach bleeding (hence its alleged safety).

Caution: Acetaminophen may also cause nausea, vomiting, chills and drowsiness. Overdoses can cause kidney or liver injury.

Products formulated specifically for menstrual and premenstrual symptoms. These products contain a unique combination of ingredients that promise to help normalize the production of prostaglandins and relax uterine muscle contractions quickly. They must be taken several times a day *before* menstruation and continued during the first few days of bleeding. These products are supposed to help curb cramps and reduce menstrual flow.

Caution: These products contain aspirin, which may cause reactions listed above; they contain caffeine which is a source of methylxanthines, said to be a factor in breast tumors, and also to blame for insomnia, nervousness and irritability. There is an aspirin-free product which contains acetaminophen (see risks above) and pamabrom, which is used to treat asthma and bronchial conditions and also has a diuretic effect; it also contains pyrilamine maleate, which is an antihistamine. (An antihistamine reaction is not part of the PMS situation, so we wonder why it is included.) These products may also cause drowsiness; they are risky for use in pregnancy or while nursing. They can also cause stomach irritation.

Ibuprofen. An analgesic or pain reliever that is said to be more effective as an anti-prostaglandin. It is said to be particularly effective for the pain of menstrual cramps. In May, 1984, the Food and Drug Administration gave approval to market ibuprofen in smaller doses as a non-prescription pain reliever. Formerly, it was available by prescription in 300-, 400- and 500-milligram doses. It will be marketed under several brand names. Ibuprofen is the first new painkiller to hit the non-prescription market since acetominophen came on the market in 1955. In this over-the-counter form, the dosage is lowered to 200 milligrams. It is said to be extremely effective in halting the action of prostaglandins and easing pain.

Caution: It is risky for aspirin-sensitive patients; it cannot be used if you have had such reactions as asthma, swelling, shock or hives. Even though this product contains no aspirin or salicylates, cross-reactions may occur in patients who are allergic to aspirin. Because it may cause heartburn, upset stomach or stomach pain, it is said to be safer if taken with food or milk. It is inadvisable for pregnant women because it may cause problems in the unborn child or complications during delivery. Ibuprofen should not be taken with other drugs; its use should be discussed with your physician. Ibuprofen should not be taken for pain for more than ten days or for fever for more than three days. Nevertheless, for many PMS sufferers, it is said to bring relief as a non-steroidal anti-prostaglandin drug.

Birth Control Pills. Oral contraceptives are said to ease distress, especially spasmodic dysmenorrhea. They prevent ovulation and hence the production of progesterone. This results in menstrual periods that are free of pain. Since there is a reduced buildup of the uterine lining, the menstrual flow is reduced; this may be the reason for less painful cramping. Theoretically, reduced hormone production prevents prostaglandin production, too.

Caution: There are many side effects with the use of the Pill. It contains progestogen (synthetic progesterone) which lowers the body's natural level and worsens an already existing estrogen/progesterone imbalance. This may exacerbate some PMS symptoms. You may have more severe headaches, depression, mood swings, fatigue, weight gain. Dr. Katharina Dalton reports that in a hospital study in which forty-four women with PMS took the Pill, forty developed side effects. She calls attention to a nation-wide English survey in which 81 percent of women with menstrual migraine said the Pill give them more painful headaches.[75]

PMS sufferers need to balance the hormones in their bodies. The Pill does the opposite by creating an *imbalance*. Some women who discontinued the Pill complained that their symptoms returned with more severity and they never could "recover."

Diuretics. You want to get rid of the bloating and water and are prescribed a diuretic. (Some are over-the-counter.) Most in use are those containing furosemide and the thiazides, especially. They do draw out excess liquids, but at a penalty.

Caution: Along with large amounts of bodily fluids drawn out by the drugs, important vitamins and minerals (especially potassium, which is needed for heart health) are also depleted. These drugs interfere with your body's natural fluid-hormonal balances, which is an undesirable reaction, since PMS is caused by an imbalance and diuretics may worsen it. You may experience dizziness, nausea, diarrhea, allergic reactions such as hives and rashes, and lightheadedness.

You may think it is safer to take a prescribed diuretic that does *not* wash potassium out of your system. This could cause an overload that may predispose to an irregular heartbeat and irritation of the gastrointestinal system. You may then have to go on a low-potassium diet which could be difficult since this heart-nourishing mineral is found in a variety of fruits and vegetables, meats and fish. You will have a hard time trying to maintain stable levels of potassium on such a program. And you are still at risk for side effects common with other diuretics. For some, even a moderate diuretic overdose can cause lethargy, weakness, excessive thirst, muscle pain and cramps.

You might do better on a salt-free diet plan that would reduce retention in your system. This would be healthier for you in the long run.

CAFFEINE + PAIN RELIEVERS

Theoretically, caffeine can boost the potency of aspirin or other pain relievers sold over the counter, say a team of researchers headed by Eugene M. Laska of the Rockland Research Institute in Orangeburg, N.Y. Some thirty pain relievers used by 10,000 patients were studied over a twenty-year span. Most of the pain relievers containing caffeine had 65 mg per tablet (130 mg per average dose).

Laska explains: "We're talking about the amount of caffeine in one or two cups of coffee. Simply drinking a cup of coffee while taking a pain reliever might not work because of other chemical constituents in the coffee." He tells of some studies showing that caffeine sped the action of the pain reliever acetaminophen by 20 to 30 percent. Most of the subjects suffered pain from uterine cramps, among other problems.

"Because most over-the-counter pain relievers can be toxic if users exceed maximum recommended doses," says William T. Beaver, M.D., of Georgetown University Schools of Medicine and Dentistry in Washington, D.C., "the findings are especially significant." He feels that caffeine could be a "safe and useful way to extend efficacy."[76]

The problem with this method is that caffeine acts as a diuretic and as a stimulant to the central nervous system. When your glands are already in turmoil and your nerves strained, to use caffeine might be pouring oil on flames.

After extensive research, specialists with the FDA did say that "when used in the recommended oral dose of 100 to 200 milligrams not more often than every three or four hours, caffeine could be safe as an analgesic adjuvant ingredient in over-the-counter menstrual drug products." But is it effective? "There is some inconclusive evidence to suggest that caffeine may exert additional analgesia (pain relief) through an adjuvant action when used in combination with other analgesics," according to the FDA.

The FDA also noted that theobromine (an alkaloid occurring in cocoa, chocolate and tea, considered similar to caffeine) "shares several pharmacological actions with . . . caffeine." *But*: "They all stimulate the central nervous system, act on the kidneys to produce diuresis, stimulate cardiac muscle and relax smooth muscle, notably bronchial muscle." Theobromine dilates coronary and other arteries; it was formerly used as a drug to treat angina. For the PMS victim, it would hardly be wise to use caffeine or theobromine for an already over-stimulated endocrine system. And you would hardly want to use a heart drug for stomach cramps.

Furthermore, since caffeine and theobromine are found in other products, you may be unaware of their buildup in your body. This overload could worsen your symptoms without your being aware of the reason. So it would make good sense to be cautious about the use of these stimulants.

Chapter 10
HERBS TO HELP "FEMALE PROBLEMS"

HERBAL or natural remedies were used for PMS back in the days when it was considered a "female problem" but before it had been identified. In modern times, we have found that herbs can be soothing and relaxing. They have been found helpful in easing spasms and contractions, as well. Many modern chemotherapeutic preparations are synthetic versions of herbs, so there is much validity in the use of these plant healers. But even though herbs are natural, many of them can cause powerful pharmacological reactions when taken in large quantities or when mixed with other ingredients. Use herbs in moderation, and follow your health professional's recommendations.

According to Mark Bricklin, author of the *Practical Encyclopedia of Natural Healing*, "Herbal tradition values several plants in assisting with problematic menstruation. Black cohosh and blue cohosh are both considered useful in expediting obstructed menstruation. They should be used moderately. A commercial product which has long been on the market contains black cohosh and a number of other herbs in an alcoholic base. The purpose of the alcohol is not simply to give the brew a zing, either. Black cohosh, like a number of other herbs, is much more soluble in alcohol than water. Little of the essence would be available from merely boiling this herb in water."

He continues, "A hot cup of ginger tea is another old standby. So are motherwort and pennyroyal. Female regulator, also known as life root and squaw weed, is considered valuable in all kinds of minor gynecological upsets. Like black cohosh, it is most soluble in alcohol.

"If you're preparing this or a similar herb at home, first boil it in water, let it cool, add some brandy, and let it stand for a few days.

"In days of yore, many herbs were prepared in this fashion and it's hard to say how much of the resulting 'relief' was from the herbs and how much from the brandy!"[77]

FOUR HERBS TO EASE PAINFUL PERIODS

To ease painful spasms, tradition suggests the use of four herbs that promise speedy relief. These are described by herbal expert Dr. Joseph Kadans, who points out that their effectiveness has been recognized for hundreds of centuries. And they are gaining new popularity in modern times, too.

1. *Balm.* Also known as sweet balm, lemon balm, garden balm or common balm. Use the dried leaves with or without the flowering tops. Just a handful of these leaves, dried or fresh, may be steeped in hot water for ten minutes and sweetened with honey to make a relaxing tea. Balm may also be taken cold by pouring a pint of boiling water over an ounce of the herb, allowing it to stand for about fifteen minutes, then letting it cool. Strain and drink freely to relieve painful periods. It has a soothing taste and fragrance like those of lemon.

2. *Black Haw*. Also known as stagbush, American sloe, viburnum, prunifolium. Use the dried bark of the root or stem. This herb acts to normalize the uterus by drawing together soft organic tissue. It protects against painful menstruation (dysmenorrhea) and also eases monthly pains, in general. Herbalists recommend one tablespoon every four hours. A pint is made by taking one ounce of the herb, soaking thoroughly in a pint of water, heated to just below the boiling point, for about fifteen minutes. Then plan to sip the recommended tablespoonful every four hours before and during the period.

3. *Ergot*. Also called ergot of rye or spurred rye. Herbalists suggest using a fluid extract. Dr. Kadans explains that ergot "has been widely used in menstrual disorders such as leucorrhea (whitish discharge from the vagina and uterine cavity), dysmenorrhea and amenorrhea (absence or abnormal stoppage of menstruation)." Dosage varies from ten to thirty drops of fluid extract.

4. *Mistletoe*. The leaves of this herb are said to act as a tonic for female ailments such as dysmenorrhea and amenorrhea. Exact dosage should be discussed with your physician.

Dr. Kadans has much praise for the use of herbs as part of a total healing program that includes the easing of PMS.[78]

MORE HERBS TO EASE MONTHLY DISTRESS

Author-researcher Dr. Jack Ritchason writes in *The Little Herb Encyclopedia*: "A female corrective herb combination will help many menstrual problems. Black cohosh is used to relieve cramps. An herbal combination for pain helps relieve the discomfort of menstrual cramps. Blue cohosh is an often used remedy to regulate the menstrual cycle."

He adds, "Muscle cramps are believed to be caused by a deficiency of calcium so a calcium-rich herb combination, alfalfa and vitamins B and E are advised. Black cohosh can cause headache if too much is used."

Dr. Ritchason suggests these herbs as part of the natural approach to relieve PMS: angelica, bayberry, bistort, blue vervain, camomile, comfrey, damiana, false unicorn, fennel, gentian, ginger, golden seal, hops, mistletoe, myrrh, parsley, peppermint, plantain, red raspberry, saffron, sage, sarsaparilla, squawvine, St. Johnswort, white oak bark, wood betony, yarrow.[79]

Herbal pharmacists and health stores that offer such a service can prepare a popular herbal combination said to help regulate hormone levels and thus relieve PMS. The combination includes the fluid extracts of: lobelia herb, meadowsweet, golden seal, red raspberry leaves, black cohosh root, marshmallow root, capsicum, ginger root.

Caution: Because each woman is different, the precise measurements should be individually prescribed by the healing specialist.

Because the pituitary gland is so closely involved in the menstrual cycle, a herbal combination that regulates this master delineator can be very welcome. The importance of this gland is cited by Frank D'Amelio, a doctor of botanical science, who explains, "The pituitary gland regulates thyroid activity, contracts blood vessels, regulates diuresis [over-secretion of urine] with vasopressin and oxytocin and regulates many other glands. It manufactures growth hormones, as well as the hormone thyrotropin which controls certain phases during pregnancy and the menstrual cycle."

To regulate the pituitary gland, Dr. D'Amelio says, "Combine the following fluid extracts: rosemary, gotu-kola, prickly ash bark, capsicum. Dose: 10-15 drops three times a day."[80] These herbs are available in liquid extract form (for speedier assimilation) at many health food stores, or at herbal practitioners.

HERBS AS DIURETICS

A well-known herbalist, Jeanne Rose, has frequently suggested the use of herbs as natural diuretics. Again, caution is the watchword since herbs can be very powerful. Always have your health practitioner regulate and prescribe dosages and formulas for your particular condition.

Jeanne Rose lists these plant products as the natural way to induce diuretic action: asparagus root, pulsatilla (also called pasque flower), which is an antispasmodic and helpful for menstrual problems, pumpkin seed, strawberry leaves, Scotch broom (seeds and twigs, sometimes used with dandelion root).

When discussing herbals with your health practitioner, ask about methods of preparation and storage and use. Since each herb is different, specific advice should be obtained.[81]

Milder Diuretics. While gentler than most herbs, these should still be used with care: dandelion tea, elder bark tea, buchu leaves tea. You may also use vegetables such as parsley, watercress, celery and cucumber. These can be part of a daily salad; they are gentle and, obviously, natural, but again, moderation is in order.

Caution: If you experience any side effects, no matter what type of diuretic or herbal product or medicine you use, it is best to stop using it. If you experience such reactions as stomach pain, nausea, unusual weakness, rapid pulse, heart palpitations, dizziness, unusual tiredness, headache, diarrhea or vomiting, it is wise to speedily discuss your reactions with your doctor. These symptoms may suggest that the product you are using is not especially suitable for your particular condition. A change may be necessary.

For general discomfort, not related to herbal or other PMS remedies, you are usually safe with a cup of herbal tea, flavored with honey and a bit of lemon. Your health store has a variety of popular teas which will help make you feel good all over, and that is just what you want to feel when in the throes of PMS.

Chapter 11
LIVING HEALTHIER
(AND HAPPIER)
WITH MENSTRUATION

EXCEPT for extreme situations, you cannot live without your monthly periods. They are a biological fact of life. But you *can* live without much of the accompanying stress and pain. By making simple adjustments in your lifestyle, you can help yourself cope with PMS and lighten the load.

Here is a set of guidelines to help you go through the cycle with a minimum of symptoms. The more closely you follow the guidelines, the better your results.

1. Warmth is comforting. It may be in the form of a hot water bottle, towel, heating pad or even a steam bath. When comfortable and doctor-approved heat is applied to the pelvic region, there is a dilation of the congested blood vessels and an easing of muscle cramps. Try warmth in other forms, too; a warm bath or shower will help your tightened muscles relax. This calms you mentally, as well. And remember hot herbal teas and caffeine-free beverages as well as hot soups but avoid sugar and salt.

2. The act of "laying on of hands" is always soothing to PMS victims. Call it massage, if you will, but the

gentle rubbing by a professional of your midsection (especially stomach) and back will relax your muscles. It is especially beneficial when a deep-heating cream or ointment is rubbed in very gently.

3. Fitness is a plus factor in your PMS-freedom program. You must exercise. No heavy barbells, though; if you try stretching and loosening-up routines, you'll open up those locked muscles. Plan to exercise from twenty to thirty minutes daily prior to, during and after your period. A good idea is to exercise all the month long to help relax your uterus and open up those rigid, taut muscles that can be cramped. Regular exercise creates a healthier blood flow that induces natural water loss, much like a diuretic. Regularly performed aerobics (jogging, swimming, stair climbing) help elevate your mood, calm you down; they act as a natural tranquilizer.

4. Oxygenate your system through deep and rhythmic breathing. In many natural childbirth classes, deep breathing is taught because it eases the pain. This same oxygenation principle helps make PMS less severe.

5. Avoid smoking. Keep away from others who smoke, as the smoke could affect your bronchial system and tighten up your circulation. This could cause more cramps. Avoid any smoke-filled area.

6. Alcohol is an iffy question. In very modest amounts, it does act as a good vasodilator; it opens up choked vessels to permit better circulation. Some specialists say that if you insist upon having that "one for the road," then you could try a 3-ounce glass of wine; or you could add a teaspoon or two of liquor to hot herbal tea. It will help buffer the onslaught of uterine-contracting prostaglandins and soothe your central nervous system. A small drink, if you must

have it, may offer a temporary relief from spasms and make you feel a bit better. See if you can do without it, though, since alcohol is not a healthful substance.

7. Get rid of the excess poundage. Overweight is one factor directly responsible for PMS. The reason is that your body's fatty tissues discharge additional estrogen which brings on the growth of the uterine lining. This can induce a heavier monthly flow. Surplus hormonal stimuli can elevate the quantity of prostaglandins released by the uterus, increasing your pain. To help control prostaglandins overload, control your appetite and weight.

8. Looking good makes you feel good. But avoid clothing that is too tight or binding, as it will hamper your circulation and worsen pelvic discomfort. No skin-tight pantyhose, girdles, jeans or tight belts.

9. Relaxation and sleep are both very effective ways of soothing menstrual pain. Try a nap. You'll awaken with less severe cramps and more energy, too. And above all, be sure to get a good night's sleep, every night. Skipping sleep builds tension and this worsens your condition. You should also take "rest breaks" throughout the day. With frequent rests, you will find it easier to cope with your condition.

10. Say "no" to salt in any form, whether from the shaker, in cooking or in packaged products. Use flavorful herbs and spices; select salt-free packaged products that are very much available in health stores and most major food stores. Always read labels.

11. Say "no" to sugar, and you can guard against overweight and the risks of hypoglycemia. A small amount of honey is permissible; use fresh fruit juices to satisfy your sweet tooth.

12. Increase your consumption of cis-linoleic acid which is found in safflower oil, especially. It initiates the formation of prostaglandin E1 (PGE1), which helps ease your PMS problems.

13. Avoid stressful situations. This can exacerbate your hypoglycemic response and worsen your symptoms. While you cannot avoid stress, you can condition yourself to avoid situations that bring on this reaction; or at least prepare to cope with them so that you do not experience excessive discomfort.

14. Your diet should emphasize complex carbohydrates; these are whole grains, fresh fruits and vegetables, legumes and beans. These will keep your blood sugar level steadier so that you avoid insulin yanks or the "yo-yo" effect caused by refined carbohydrates. Try cheese, yogurt (salt and sugar free, please), nuts, sunflower seeds, popcorn (salt and oil free).

15. Granted that PMS is a personal matter, you may need to explain it to people with whom you come in contact, whether at home, at work, at school or anywhere else. A few words to just one or two understanding people will make life easier for everyone.

Let's look at three categories which include most women and see how to avoid conflicts and manage to stay in good mental and physical shape with a sensible attitude.

THE PMS "AT-HOME" WOMAN

You do have an advantage over working women in that you can be at home most of the time, but you could have problems with your husband and/or children. And you can have extra difficulties if you drag yourself around the house, moping and feeling sorry for yourself.

Instead, try to follow a schedule. *Give yourself time*

for all of your daily activities. No rushing—but do not let yourself become semi-comatose when you awaken. Sure, give yourself a few moments to wake up. Get your thoughts and muscles in order. But plan to go about your activities before too long.

Make yourself look reasonably pretty, even if you are staying at home. A frilly garment, a fragrance, a bold makeup color will all brighten up your mood.

Tidy up the house. Do necessary cleaning. If you have a mate and/or children, plan for their arrival that evening. Straighten up their rooms, too. Make certain everything is as much in order as it is comfortably possible to do so. Your "blue moods" will brighten up when you do things for others. You will help get your mind off yourself.

If you feel all tied up in knots, you can still manage to do your household activities. Do only the necessities like cleaning up and preparing the evening meal. No heavy housework if you are heavy with PMS.

Outside appointments with the beautician, dentist, manicurist or what-have-you can be postponed for a better time, but only if you feel you cannot manage. It might help cheer you up to be with others.

Never, but never, just lie around the house and commiserate with yourself. Do not loll in bed. You become stagnant. Your mental outlook is foggy. You need to keep reasonably active.

Be sure to observe the six-meals-a-day program. A high complex carbohydrate breakfast is a must plus frequent snacks of low-calorie vegetables, and a good lunch and dinner with several smaller mini-meals. But remember, the meals should be nourishing and within caloric limits. Take time for exercise at home, too. Just thirty minutes can help loosen up any tightness.

Explain to your husband that you are in the midst of

PMS. If you live with other relations, let them know, also. This can work wonders in helping them understand your reactions, sympathize with you, offer you help when needed.

It is also helpful to talk your problems over with a sympathetic listener—a social worker, clergyman, doctor, relative, close friend or anyone who can understand what you are going through. Talking over your fears can help allay them and this is important if you are alone during the day.

Do not isolate yourself, though. A walk to a nearby park is helpful. Visit a local recreational affair. Eat lunch in a quiet square. Visit shops and museums. Whatever keeps you active, does not cause strain, helps take your mind off PMS will be a good health tonic. Aim for a balance between household routine and recreation, with and without your family, and you should be able to better withstand your symptoms.

THE PMS WORKING WOMAN

You may feel like a martyr in the morning, if you have to go to work with PMS. Plan ahead. If you experience excruciating pain, then it would be best to telephone your supervisor and remain home. After all, you do have responsibilities on the job and you cannot fulfill them if you are sick. If you can cope with your responsibilities, then go ahead.

Transportation should be carefully considered if you are experiencing severe symptoms. Severe headaches, drug reactions or emotional upset could make you a high-risk driver. It would be best to use mass transportation or leave the driving to someone else.

Do NOT neglect the rules about diet, even if you have to work. A good breakfast, some fresh fruit, a glass of mineral water will help raise your blood sugar levels.

And plan to eat nourishing foods at a restaurant during the workday, too. Not available? Then brown bag it!

Take time to make yourself look attractive. If need be, disguise any bloating with the proper clothes. It is important to make yourself look attractive. You will find that it lifts your spirits.

Before you leave for work, about ten or fifteen minutes of exercise will help loosen up any tightness. It helps whip up your sluggish circulation and clear the cobwebs from your mind. You'll then be better able to face your responsibilities.

Be prepared for some stress on the job. Rare is the workday without some problems. If you have unusual symptoms, confide to an understanding supervisor. Postpone any important meetings. Plan to reduce your workload. Again, you need the cooperation of your superior. Any serious decisions should also be delayed until the cycle has ended.

A PMS "first-aid" kit should be with you at your desk or in your handbag. This can include such items as vegetable chunks prepared early in the morning; chunks of salt-free cheese; small cubes of leftover beef; a chicken or turkey drumstick; herbal teabags; salt-free soup cubes; wholegrain crackers (salt and sugar free); an apple, pear or banana; nuts and seeds. Remember, you do not want to let yourself get hungry; a growling stomach can trigger off serious reactions. Since you are on the job, you can't easily run out or to your refrigerator for food. You need it at hand. A comfortably hot beverage is also soothing.

Schedule your chores so that you can perform diligently but not to the point of exhaustion. It is best to go outdoors during your lunch period. A brief walk in the fresh air and sunshine will help make you feel better. A change of scenery will wipe away fatigue and give you a lift.

Have a "coffee break"? No caffeine beverages, as you already know. Why not try meditation? Relax. Close your eyes. Breathe deeply, in and out. Visualize the starry heavens, the multi-colored gardens of a fantastic castle, the glittering seashore, the brightness of a rainbow. Just let your thoughts soar upward and outward. Contemplate the wondrous immensity of the universe. After just fifteen minutes, you will feel as refreshed as if you had ventured to the outer limits of the stratosphere and then returned again.

Back at work, try to avoid any heavy or unpleasant chores. They could worsen your condition. Again, establish rapport with your superior and explain the situation. You do want to do your share, but during these few days, you prefer activities that are consistent with your condition. You should be able to fulfill your obligations with an understanding superior.

At home, pamper yourself. Take care of obligations to others, then just relax. It will ease the day's stress, make it easier for you to sleep at night and then help you face tomorrow's workday.

THE PMS SCHOOLGIRL

If you are a schoolgirl suffering from PMS, you need to reconcile yourself to the situation. But don't just suffer . . . do something!

It is, of course, essential for you to have a calendar or chart. You will then be able to know when the time is approaching. Explain it to your family. Yes, you may feel shy, unsure of yourself, but just suffering in silence will make it worse for you. It will help matters if you prepare for the situation and deal with it head on.

Many teenage girls are embarrassed by tender breasts.

Wear a more accommodating bra; if need be, discuss it with your family physician. Up tight about a male doctor? Then find a woman physician if it will make you more comfortable. Ask about emotional upsets and how to control them. Just talking can help allay your fears.

Expect some weight gain because of fluid retention. Do not be frightened by the scales. When the cycle is over, you will lose water and the weight. If you use the menstrual chart properly, you will note there is a corresponding reduction in the amount of urine passed in the early days of the cycle. It is being stored, and will be eliminated when the cycle is over.

Teenagers during PMS seem to be hardest hit in terms of abnormal food urges. Hormonal changes, a deficiency of essential fatty acids and water displacement can all give you such cravings. If you give in to rich and fattening junk foods, you will be vulnerable to weight gain, as well as to an imbalance in blood sugar.

To counteract, have a healthy breakfast. Take a healthy lunch with you, too. And remember, include some high protein, high complex carbohydrate snacks as suggested above to help calm down acute hunger pangs. Chomp away on raw vegetables instead of gulping down sugary soda drinks or candy bars. Thirsty? Try a glass of skim milk or a fruit juice that is sugar-free.

You may also note swelling of fingers, wrists, ankles and stomach. If rings, bracelets, watch straps are too tight, if shoes are uncomfortable, make some changes. Clothes can be adjusted to accommodate the bulge. Avoid jewelry. After a few days, you should be all right again.

Try to make school as easy for yourself as possible. Granted that you cannot tell your teacher to postpone an exam, but if you have other obligations that may be trying for you, explain that you are not feeling well and ask if they may be postponed. A talk with your school nurse or teacher, should help straighten out problems.

Feel lethargic? Unable to concentrate? Feel fidgety during an examination? Prepare for these possibilities by getting enough sleep the night before, good food during the day, enough outdoor exercise or activity so that you will be refreshed. If at all possible, try to get major projects taken care of prior to the onset of your symptoms. If you follow the guidelines given throughout this book, you should have more physical and mental energy than ordinary and be equal to the tasks at hand.

FEELING BETTER NOW?

With the mysteries dispelled and with greater understanding of your body, you should feel better knowing that you can do something about menstrual discomforts.

Great-grandmother may have said she "fell off the roof." Grandmother sometimes called it "the curse." Mother referred to it as her "time of the month." For generations spoken of in euphemisms and cloaked in myth and superstition, menstruation is now openly discussed, often quite loudly, in the news media and at home.

Modern medicine and psychology are chipping away at the myths surrounding menstruation. They are providing a scientific basis for the treatment of PMS that will help you have healthy, trouble-free reproductive years. With better self-care and the use of nutrition, fitness and modern methods of pain relief, you can start feeling better soon—maybe even next month.

References

1. Niels H. Lauersen, M.D., *Premenstrual Syndrome and You* (New York, N.Y.: Fireside Books, Simon & Schuster, Inc., 1983), 33.
2. Caroline Shreeve, M.D., *The Premenstrual Syndrome* (Wellingborough, Northamptonshire, England: Thorsons Publishers Ltd., 1983).
3. Simone de Beauvoir, *The Second Sex* (New York, N.Y.: Alfred A. Knopf, 1952).
4. Ronald V. Norris, M.D., *PMS: Premenstrual Syndrome* (New York, N.Y.: Rawson Associates, 1983).
5. Sheila MacLeod, *The Art of Starvation* (New York, N.Y.: Schocken Books, 1982).
6. Robert T. Frank, M.D., "Hormonal Causes of Premenstrual Tension," *Archives of Neurology and Psychiatry* (1931): 26:1053.
7. Harvey E. Billig, Jr., M.D. and S. Arthur Spaulding, Jr., M.D., "Hyperinsulinism of Menses," *Industrial Medicine* (July, 1947): 336-339.
8. Katharina Dalton, M.D., and Raymond Greene, "The Premenstrual Syndrome," *British Medical Journal* (May 9, 1953), 1007-1016.
9. "Dysmenorrhea and Premenstrual Syndrome." National Institutes of Health, Bethesda, Maryland, 1983.
10. Katharina Dalton, M.D., *Once a Month. The Premenstrual Syndrome: What it is and How to Free Yourself from its Effects* (Pomona, California: Hunter House, 1979).
11. Arianna Stassinopoulos, *Maria Callas* (New York, N.Y.: Ballantine Books, 1982).

12. Christopher Finch, *Rainbow* (New York, N.Y.: Grosset & Dunlap, 1975).

13. Christine Crawford, *Mommie Dearest* (New York, N.Y.: Berkley Books, 1981).

14. W. A. Evans, *Mrs. Abraham Lincoln—A Study of Her Personality and Her Influence on Lincoln* (New York, N.Y.: Alfred A. Knopf, 1932).

15. Sylvia Plath, *The Journals of Sylvia Plath* (New York, N.Y.: Dial Press, 1982).

16. Brooks Ranney, M.D., "Premenstrual Tension," press release, American College of Obstetricians and Gynecologists, May 24, 1982.

17. Neils H. Lauersen, M.D., and Zoe R. Graves, Ph.D., "A New Approach to Premenstrual Syndrome," *The Female Patient*, Vol. 8 (April 1983): 41-54.

18. News release, New York, N.Y.: Medical and Pharmaceutical Information Bureau, Inc., August 17, 1982.

19. News release, "The Growth of Sexual Medicine," The Upjohn Company, April 2, 1984.

20. Timothy Johnson, M.D., *The Harvard Medical School Health Letter Book* (New York, N.Y., Warner Books, 1981).

21. *USA Today*, March 15, 1984.

22. "Dysmenorrhea and Premenstrual Syndrome," National Institutes of Health, Bethesda, Maryland, 1983.

23. Dalton, *Once a Month*.

24. Norris, *PMS*.

25. Katharina Dalton, M.D., "Menstruation and Crime," *British Medical Journal*, 2:1752.

26. Morton S. Biskind, M.D., "Nutritional Deficiency in the Etiology of Menorrhagia, Metrohagia, Cystic Mastitis and Premenstrual Tension, Treatment with Vitamin B Complex," *Journal of Clinical Endocrinology and Metabolism*, 3 (1943): 227-234.

27. Guy E. Abraham, M.D., *Premenstrual Blues* (Torrance, California: Optimox Corporation, 1980), 15.

28. Patricia Allen, M.D., and Denise Fortino, *Cycles: Every Woman's Guide to Menstruation* (New York, N.Y., Pinnacle Books, 1983), 147.

29. Emrika Padus, *Woman's Encyclopedia of Health and Natural Healing* (Emmaus, Pa.: Rodale Press, 1981), 382-383.

30. Family Practice News, Washington, D.C., March 14, 1974.

31. R. S. London, M.D., "Premenstrual Symptoms," *The Journal of the American College of Nutrition*, 2 (1983): 115-122.

32. John Ellis, M.D. *Vitamin B6, The Doctor's Report* (New York, N.Y.: Harper & Row, 1973).

33. Barbara Seaman and Gideon Seaman, M.D., *Women and the Crisis in Sex Hormones* (New York, N.Y.: Bantam Books, Inc., 1978).

34. International Medical News Service, Washington, D.C., press release, February, 1984.

35. Mona M. Shangold, M.D., "Drug Therapy for the Premenstrual Syndrome," *The Journal of Reproductive Medicine*, Vol. 28, No. 7 (1983).

36. Guy E. Abraham, M.D., and J. Hargrove, M.D., "Effect of Vitamin B6 on infertility in Women with the Premenstrual Tension Syndrome," *Infertility*, 2 (1979):315.

37. T. McKenna, M.D., D. Island, M.D., W. Nicholson, M.D., "Dopamine Inhibits Angiotensin-Stimulated Aldosterone Biosynthesis in Bovine Adrenal Cells." *Journal of Clinical Investigation*, 64 (1979):287.

38. H. Schaumburg, M.D., J. Kaplan, M.D., S. Rasmus, M.D., "Pyridoxine Megavitaminosis Produces Sensory Neuropathy In Humans," *Annals of Neurology*, 12 (1982):107-8.

39. Lauersen, *PMS*.

40. Guy E. Abraham, M.D., M. M. Lubran, M.D., "Serum and Red Cell Magnesium Levels in Patients with Premenstrual Tension," *American Journal of Clinical Nutrition*, 34 (1981):2364.

41. Bernard Horn, M.D., quoted in *Prevention* magazine, November, 1982, 145-146.

42. Guy E. Abraham, M.D., et al., "Effect of Vitamin B6 on Plasma and Red Blood Cell Magnesium Levels in Premenopausal Women," *American Journal of Clinical Laboratory Science*, 11 (1981):333.

43. Lauersen, *PMS*.

44. Jane Brody, *Jane Brody's Nutrition Book* (New York, N.Y.: Bantam Books, 1982), 128.

45. Lauersen, *"A New Approach."*

46. Norris, *PMS*.

47. Dalton, *"Once a Month."*

48. Science News, *"Premenstrual Changes,"* Vol. 122 (December 11, 1982), 380-381.

49. Allen, *Cycles*, 77
50. Michael G. Brush, M.D., and Judy Lever, *Premenstrual Tension* (New York, N.Y.: McGraw-Hill Book Company), 39-40.
51. Jennifer Allen, "*Premenstrual Frenzy*," *New York* magazine (November 1, 1982), 37-42.
52. Lauersen, *PMS*.
53. S. Simkins, M.D., "Use of massive doses of Vitamin A in the treatment of hyperthyroidism," *Journal of Clinical Endocrinological Metabolism* 7 (1947):572.
54. *Woman's Encyclopedia of Health and Natural Healing* (Emmaus, Pa.: Rodale Press, Inc., 1981).
55. Ellis, *Vitamin B6*.
56. Evan Shute, M.D., *Vitamin E* (London, Ontario, Canada: Shute Brothers Clinic, 1969).
57. Lauersen, *PMS*.
58. "How To Deal With Your Tensions" (Arlington, Virginia: National Mental Health Association, 1981).
59. *Physical Fitness Research Digest* (Washington, D.C.: President's Council on Physical Fitness, July, 1978).
60. Penny Wise Budoff, *No More Menstrual Cramps and Other Good News* (New York, N.Y.: Penguin Books, 1981).
61. Lauersen, *PMS*, 83.
62. W. Y. Chan, M.D., M. Y. Dawood, M.D., F. Fuchs, M.D., "Relief of Dysmenorrhea with the Prostaglandin Synthetase Inhibitor Ibuprofen: Effect on Prostaglandin Levels in Menstrual Fluid," *American Journal of Obstetrics and Gynecology* 135 (1, 1979):102-108.
63. Shreeve, *Premenstrual Syndrome*.
64. David Horrobin, M.D., "Actions of Prolactin on Human Renal Function," *Lancet*, 2 (1971):352.
65. David F. Horrobin, M.D., *Medical Hypotheses* 6 (1980): 785-800.
66. M. Moore, *Medicinal Herbs of the West* (Albuquerque, New Mexico: University of New Mexico Press, 1979).
67. David F. Horrobin, M.D. *Medical Hypotheses* 5 (1979): 969-985.
68. Lauersen, *PMS*.
69. Horrobin, *See note 65*.
70. M. G. Brush, M.D. "Therapy for the Woman with Premenstrual Syndrome," *Mims* (April 1, 1982), 7-31.

71. Horrobin, *See note 63*.
72. "What About Evening Primrose Oil?" *Spring* Magazine (October, 1983), 22.
73. *Ibid*.
74. Dianne Hales, "Flower Power: Evening Primrose Oil" *Redbook* magazine (July, 1983), 29-30.
75. Dalton, *Once a Month*.
76. *Journal of the American Medical Association*, as quoted in *The New York Times*, April 6, 1984.
77. Mark Bricklin, *Practical Encyclopedia Of Natural Healing* (Emmaus, Penna.: Rodale Press, 1976).
78. Joseph Kadans, *Encyclopedia of Medicinal Herbs* (West Nyack, N.Y.: Parker Publishing Co., Inc. 1970).
79. Dr. Jack Ritchason, *The Little Herb Encyclopedia* (Springville, Utah: Thornwood Books, 1980).
80. Dr. Frank D'Amelio, *The Botanical Practitioner* (Bellmore, N.Y.,: Holistic Publishing Co., 1982).
81. Jeanne Rose, *Herbs & Things* (New York, N.Y.: Grosset & Dunlap, 1972).

The Best in Health Books by
LINDA CLARK,
BEATRICE TRUM HUNTER
and CARLSON WADE

By Linda Clark

☐ **Know Your Nutrition** — $4.95
☐ **Face Improvement Through Nutrition** — $2.25
☐ **Be Slim and Healthy** — $1.50
☐ **Go-Caution-Stop Carbohydrate Computer** — $1.95
☐ **The Best of Linda Clark** — $4.50
☐ **How to Improve Your Health** — $4.95

By Beatrice Trum Hunter

☐ **Whole Grain Baking Sampler**
    ☐ Cloth $6.95   ☐ Paperback $2.95
☐ **Additives Book** — $2.25
☐ **Fermented Foods and Beverages** — $1.25
☐ **Yogurt, Kefir & Other Milk Cultures** — $1.75
☐ **Wheat, Millet and Other Grains** — $1.45
☐ **High Power Foods** — $1.45

By Carlson Wade

☐ **Arthritis and Nutrition** — $1.95
☐ **Bee Pollen** — $2.50
☐ **Lecithin** — $2.25
☐ **Fats, Oils and Cholesterol** — $1.50
☐ **Vitamins and Other Supplements** — $1.50
☐ **Hypertension (High Blood Pressure) and Your Diet** — $1.95

Buy them at your local health or book store or use this coupon.

Keats Publishing, Inc. (P.O. Box 876), New Canaan, Conn. 06840
Please send me the books I have checked above. I am enclosing
$_____ (add $1.00 to cover postage and handling). Send check
or money order — no cash or C.O.D.'s please.

Mr/Mrs/Miss _____

Address_____

City_____State_____Zip_____
(Allow three weeks for delivery)